fastrack to wellness
good health. good life. guide

First Edition

Designed by Piret Mikk/Inox DM

Printed by CreateSpace, An Amazon.com Company
To contact the author, visit www.fastrackwellness.com
ISBN-10: 0990859401
ISBN-13: 978-0-9908594-0-6
Self-Help, Motivational & Inspirational

fastrack to wellness
good health. good life. guide

by helen marie loorents

I am dedicating this book to all the busy professionals in the world who are overwhelmed by their lives and are looking for ways to improve their health and well-being. Whether it is finding work-life balance, relief from stress and anxiety, more energy and increased productivity, managing weight or, most important, having good relationships and love, this book can help you.

You can have it all! There is a simple way to good health and good life that fits into your busy lifestyle. This book is about you, your health and your life.

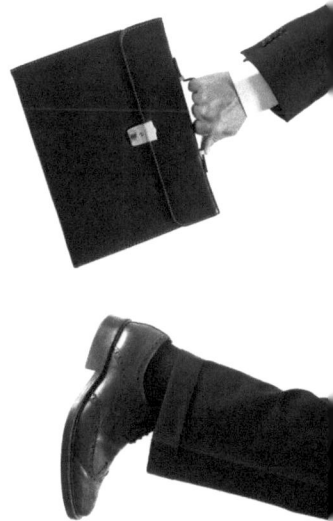

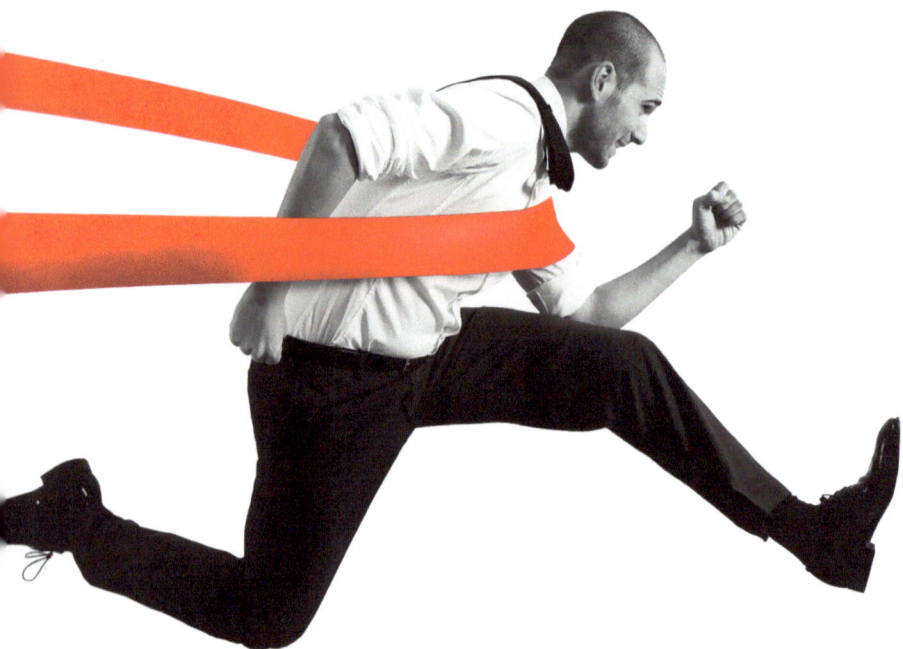

contents

acknowledgments

First, I would like to acknowledge my dad, who was my first client and who truly transformed his life within five (5) months. He followed my guidance even during times when it was difficult for him. He began his life-altering journey as a grumpy old man, 30 pounds overweight, on high blood pressure medication, who had difficulty walking a few feet, and couldn't tie his own shoelaces. Five months later, he is exactly as he used to be 20 years ago. He now is a youthful, fun, smart, optimistic, energetic, athletic man whom my mom married 38 years ago, and the amazing man my family has always known. I also see my dad as a torture test because, if I can help change a stubborn, "my way or the highway," proud, super-confident, successful man, I can help change anybody!

I would like to give special thanks to my mom, who has always been there for me, for better or worse. There was a time when she was the only person who believed in me and encouraged me to stay on the course to make my dreams come true. Without that encouragement and support, I wouldn't be where I am today and you wouldn't be reading this book.

I also would like to acknowledge my former employers, GlaxoSmithKline, Johnson & Johnson, and Colgate Palmolive. I wouldn't be able to write this book without that corporate experience.

I am grateful to Joshua Rosenthal, the founder and director of the Institute for Integrative Nutrition. The health-coaching program there is topnotch and his inspiration and guidance have been life-changing.

Special thanks to my editor, Mila Andre, who made sure the information herein is understood by all.

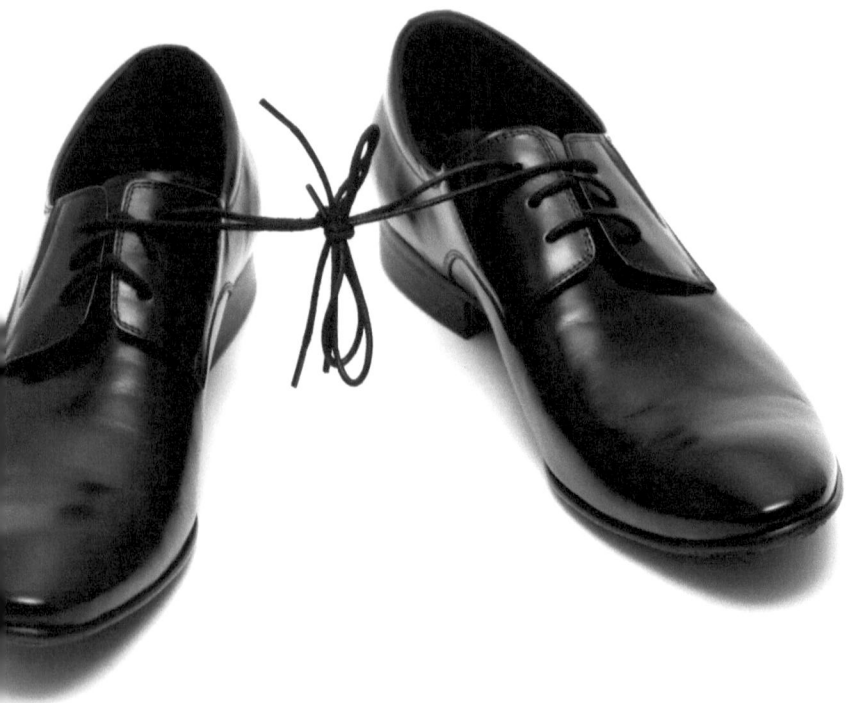

introduction

Welcome to the "fastrack to wellness" guide! This guide has been written with the intent to help transform lives of busy professionals by helping each individual achieve "good health. good life." in a fast, simple way. I know you have no time, that's why I am here to share with you everything you need to know about "good health. good life." in a holistic way, so you can be healthy and happy.

- Do you feel like there are not enough hours in a day?
- Feeling stressed out?
- Do you not like what you see in the mirror?
- Feel like you could improve your personal life?
- Do you want more energy and be more productive?
- Is your body telling you it is time to rest?
- Are you living a life you were meant to be living?
- Do you want to be healthier and happier but find it overwhelming?

There are thousands of books, newsletters, articles, training sessions, doctors and boot camps for every part of your body, and sometimes they contradict each other.

If you answered YES to any of the above, then you are at the right place at the right time.

I am Helen Marie Loorents, founder and CEO of **fastrack wellness inc.**, certified health & life coach, corporate wellness expert, Reiki master-energy healer, yoga instructor, published author and speaker. And also a former corporate marketing executive with an MBA.

Exactly a year ago, September 2013, I walked away from a 17-year-long successful career working for big corporations like Colgate Palmolive, Johnson & Johnson, and GlaxoSmithKline. I walked away because I got totally burnt out, my body hurt all over and I was unhappy. Yes, I did live on Wall St. in a fancy apartment and drove a Lexus, but none of those material things brought me happiness. I didn't know what to do next, but I knew what I was doing was not working for me. I took a year off. I traveled around the world, mastering health and life. And spent time with my family in stillness, peace and quiet – the only way true healing can occur.

I started the company because I was seeing many busy professionals around me being exactly at the same place where I used to be – they have a lot of success in their lives but they are unhappy and a majority of them are unhealthy. Something always is missing and everything looks a lot better from the outside than inside. Why is it that many people who are well off are not happy? How should we live our lives so we can be healthy and happy? That became the purpose of my journey – discovering simple truths behind "good health. good life."

After traveling the world, studying and learning everything that interests me, spending time in stillness and becoming a Reiki master, my vision became so clear that I am now actually able to see that purple third eye, called intuition. It has been guiding me ever since and that's how I came up with the idea to write this book. Now don't get intimidated by this third eye stuff, because we all have it; we just have gotten too involved in the hustle and bustle of life and have lost touch with ourselves as well as the world around us. Regardless, the third eye, your intuition, is still there and is guiding you every step of the way. Most of us experience bumps in the road because that's the way your inner guidance tries to correct your actions, your life.

It is my mission to pass on a simple holistic view of the "good health. good life." guide to all of those busy professionals who are looking to be healthy and happy in life but have no time to research the Internet, attend days-long training classes nor read thousands of books about body, mind and spirit. I want to transfer all my fast, easy, simple wellness techniques – that I mastered in a few years – to all of you, so you can start living a healthy, happy life now. Also, the information in this book is for corporations and businesses to implement, because the greatest asset to a company is a healthy, happy employee. That positive energy and increased productivity will make the company blossom.

When I started **fastrack wellness inc.**, I was a little hesitant because I only have a few years' worth of health and wellness expertise. Okay, it helps that I am a European and always have been into healthy eating and yoga, but that's about it. So how can I compete with experts who have doctorates in psychology, fitness, and nutrition, and have 40 years under their belts. Then, I realized, this is it! I've been on the other side with all of you, working 24/7 for 17 years and know exactly what you are going through and what you need. I have also mastered quick techniques to transform my own health and life in a very short period of time, as well as transforming the lives of others, and now I can pass it on to the world.

You do not need a PhD in health and wellness, nor do you need years of healthy habits; all you need is to take the first step now and your life will change. It's fast, easy and simple, but you do need to be ready to do the work. According to the study published in the European Journal of Social Psychology in 2010[1], it took people 18 to 254 days to change to a new health-related habit, as it varies from person to person how long it takes to "rewire" the neural network in our brain. We have to slowly learn a new habit and replace the old one with it. That takes time and repetition. Plus, remember, we have busy jobs, so all this new stuff needs to work with our busy lifestyle. We also know "easy come, easy go." So when it comes to modifying a lifestyle, the behavioral changes must be gradual, systematic and non-invasive. We need to love those changes in order to stick to them. The 5-month program has been proven to work for most people, but it does vary depending on how long you have been practicing bad habits and how open you are to change.

Our life, our health are like a golf game; we need the right TECHNIQUE and PRACTICE in order to win. Without those two, it really comes down to luck. The same applies to "good health. good life." We need to learn the right TECHNIQUE and then we need to PRACTICE it consistently in order to succeed. At the same time, we all are unique and have our incredible talents and gifts. We all need to polish different parts of the game. Thus, the winning formula of "good health. good life." is different for each of us.

All golfers hire coaches to learn to play golf, but we often take good health, good life for granted and assume it comes naturally. Perhaps it did thousands of years ago because we were very much connected with our intuition and our environment. Technology has taken over and now we trust Google more than our own inner guidance. We have lost the ability to trust ourselves, and our faith is weaker than ever before. But there is no reason to get discouraged, because "good health. good life." is so simple that anyone can master it; so let's get right to it.

This book is all about "good health. good life." TECHNIQUE. PRACTICE is left for each individual to carry out through PRACTICAL TOOLS. The latter is most important because we have all the health and wellness information now readily available to us, but how often do we really use it to change our behavior, our lives? Reading alone is not going to lead to behavior change. A new, different action will lead to a behavior change. To paraphrase Albert Einstein, "If you keep doing the same thing over and over again expecting a different outcome, you must be insane."

The "fastrack to wellness" guide has 7 "good health. good life." MODULES. The reason we need to address both life and health is that they are inherently connected. What goes on in your head, your emotions, directly impacts your physical body, your health. Thus, to achieve optimum health and well-being, we cannot separate them.

There is nothing more important than your health and your life, so let's PRACTICE living a good life. Those PRACTICAL TOOLS are important because, as stated before, we are all unique. We all have different backgrounds, issues, challenges, limiting beliefs, blocks, fears, dietary restrictions, body types, blood types, fitness levels, preferences, etc. Not one solution will work for everybody. We need to address them individually so we can truly transform our lives. This book will guide you to create your own winning formula for "good health. good life."

Now, let's get started!

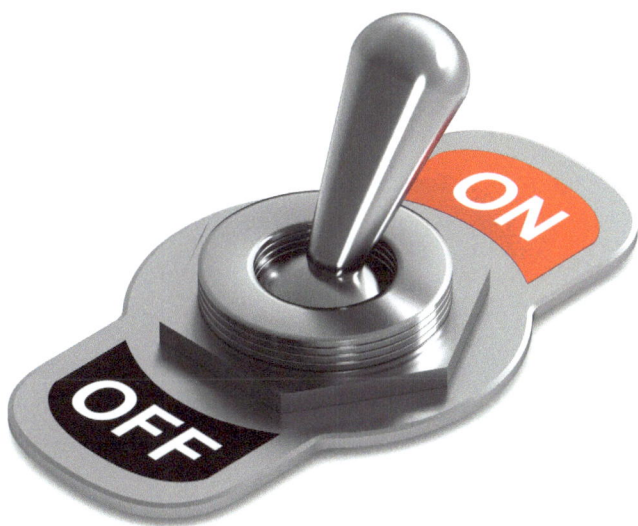

overview - the winning formula

If I were to ask you what prevents you from getting everything you ever wanted, you would probably tell me it is TIME. Time is precious and, as J.R.R. Tolkien said, "All we have to decide is what to do with the time that is given us." We busy professionals have no TIME, so we need things that are fast, easy, simple and effective, otherwise we just won't do them.

- Would you eat healthy if you could learn how to cook healthy meals in 15 minutes, and lose weight?
- Would you exercise more if you could burn as many calories within 20 minutes as you would normally within 60 minutes?
- Would you meditate if you could do a 1½-minute breathing exercise twice a day that would make you fall asleep like a baby, drop your blood pressure and open your mind to new possibilities?

The fastrack to wellness winning formula is simple. There are three layers to "good health. good life." and they are interconnected:
1. good mind
2. good body
3. good emotions

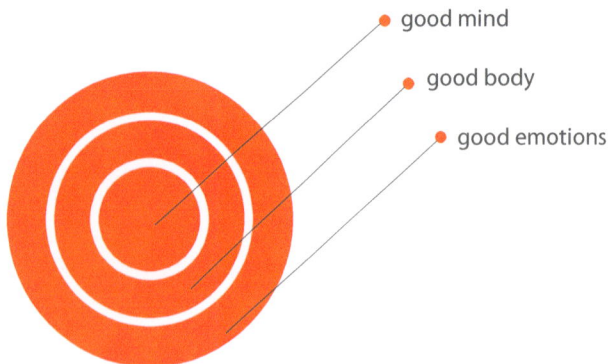

- good mind
- good body
- good emotions

It all starts from the inside out. You can read "The Secret," by Rhonda Byrne; "The Law of Attraction: The Basics of the Teaching of Abraham," by Esther Hicks and Jerry Hicks; "The Art of Happiness, 10ᵗʰ Anniversary Edition: A Handbook for Living," by Dalai Lama; "The Heart of the Buddha's Teaching: Transforming Suffering Into Peace, Joy, and Liberation," by Thich Nhat Hanh or even the Bible; it all comes back to, "What I give out is what I get back. What I believe in, becomes true for me."

Your life is a reflection of who you are. Your thoughts, beliefs, values and actions define your reality and perception. Focus on the inside. Once you get the THOUGHTS right, the outside takes care of itself. In other words, the inner balance leads to outer balance. This is the only way to true happiness; there is no other way. You can be on a healthy diet and exercise all you want, but your mind drives your state of happiness. Your mind drives how beautiful you look and if you are able to lose those last 5 pounds. So now you probably are thinking, "How can I possibly change the inside, the mind?" Not to worry; there are simple techniques to incorporate into your daily life, and the changes are transformational.

Our 7 MODULES will summarize everything you need to know about "good health. good life." We will cover "good mind" in **MODULES 1-3**:

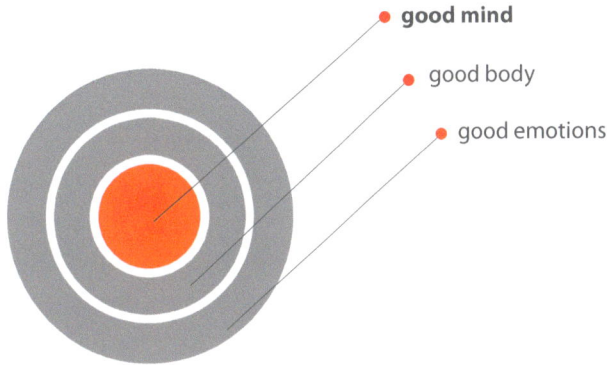

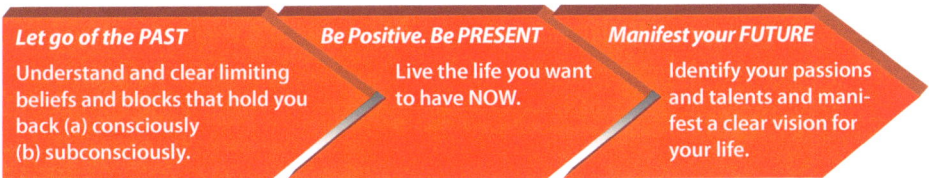

good mind

good body

good emotions

Let go of the PAST
Understand and clear limiting beliefs and blocks that hold you back (a) consciously (b) subconsciously.

Be Positive. Be PRESENT
Live the life you want to have NOW.

Manifest your FUTURE
Identify your passions and talents and manifest a clear vision for your life.

To sum this up, the first step is to truly understand our values and beliefs, and especially the limiting ones that have held us back. Perhaps we think, "If I lose those 15 pounds, then I will be beautiful." or, "When I get that new job, then I will be happy." In reality, once we get those things, then we want to lose another 5 pounds and need to get another promotion, and the target keeps moving further away and so does the state of happiness.

How do we break that pattern? More to come in Module 1. We all know we only use 10% of our brain (the conscious part) and 90% is unused. This is where the subconscious kicks in and often does more of the work without us even knowing it. It is important to clear all the brain of all the limitations so we can truly flourish and have the abundance we are seeking.

The second step is to live in the present moment, because that is all that's guaranteed to us. We often worry about the past and the future, and truly miss the present. One of the models to help us live a "good life" is called the BE-DO-HAVE model, which some say was first introduced by L. Ron Hubbard in his book, "Conditions of Existence." The model guides us to focus on the now: "Based on what do I want to BE, I do the things I need to DO, and the result is that I HAVE what I want." Every thought, every word, every action creates your life. Like Mahatma Gandhi said, "Be the change that you wish to see in the world."

The last part of "good mind" is manifesting our FUTURE. This seems quite obvious, but most of us never get to that stillness, the peace and quiet to truly figure out what we really do want in life. What are our true passions, talents – things that come easily to us? We often keep doing the same thing and expecting a different outcome. Our mind is like a GPS. It tells the body, the universe, which way we want to go. If we signal different messages and are not quite sure where we want to go, we will never reach the destination, but will keep going around in circles.

We will spend **MODULES 4-6** on "good body" and there is a lot to cover, starting with nutrition and ending with fitness, sleep leading to energy and looking good.

good mind

good body

good emotions

You are what you EAT	MOVE & SLEEP for energy	LOOK good
Your food is your medicine.	Move 30 minutes every day & sleep so you have the energy you need.	Be beautiful inside and out.

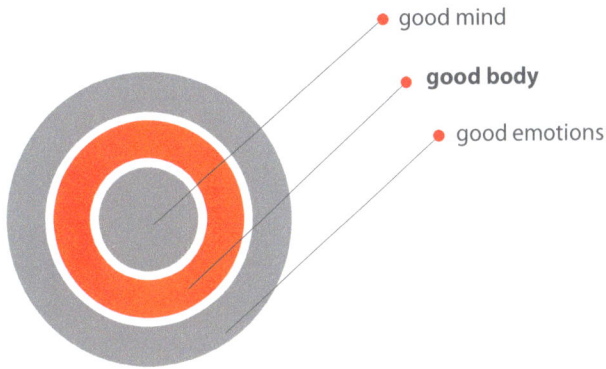

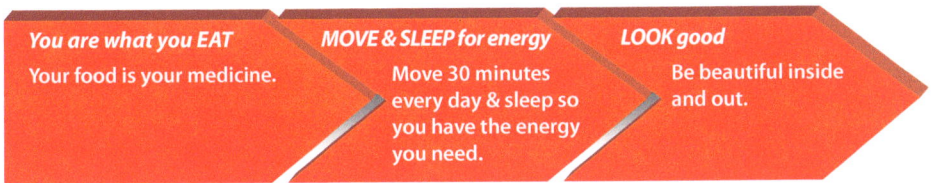

Our food is our medicine, so we do need to listen to our body to figure out what we need, what satisfies us and what leaves us empty and unfulfilled. This depends on so many things: your blood type, your heritage, your geography, climate, lifestyle. There is no one diet that works for everybody. And, by the way, how many diets have you tried? We will discover how we break free from that pattern of yo-yo dieting and enter a lifestyle of food for energy and nutrition.

We do know we are meant to be moving every day and it doesn't have to be going to the gym five times a week. We often push ourselves to the limit and that's when our bodies start telling us, "Slow down," as we ache all over. Or we're in pain when we don't exercise. It all has to be in perfect balance. Listen to your body and it will tell you what it needs. Take a break and rest when your body demands it. This is equally important to moving your body.

We are also meant to be sleeping for 7 to 8 hours. Most of us are lucky if we get 5-6 hours of sleep. It may be productive for a short period of time, as the adrenalin keeps us going, but then it catches us off-guard. At that point, most likely we are calling in sick because we can't get out of bed and all we want is to sleep. We will talk about that super-effective 1½-minute breathing exercise in this section. You probably will sleep like a baby!

The last part of "good body" is "look good." We live in a physical world and like attracts like. So be the person whom you want to meet or people with whom you want to hang out. As we start becoming clear about who we are, our identity, what drives us, what makes us happy, we will start seeing ourselves in a different light. We may recognize, at this point, that it is time for a makeover because the old no longer serves the new identity. Remember, our perspective creates our reality, so if our perspectives are changing, be ready for the reality to change as well. At this time, many of you will look at your wardrobes and say, "What was I thinking?"

We will cover "good emotions" in **MODULE 7.**

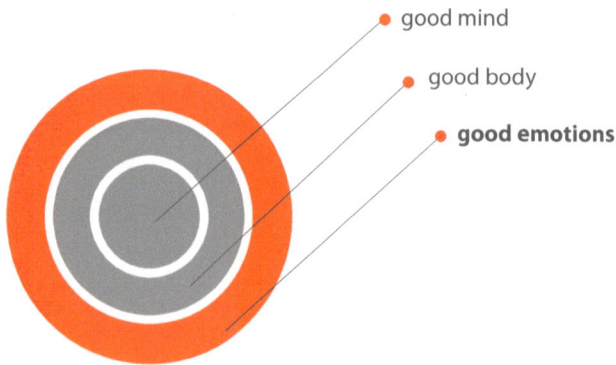

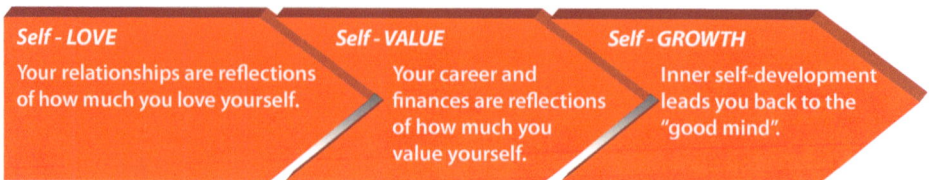

- good mind
- good body
- **good emotions**

Self - LOVE
Your relationships are reflections of how much you love yourself.

Self - VALUE
Your career and finances are reflections of how much you value yourself.

Self - GROWTH
Inner self-development leads you back to the "good mind".

"If you want
something you've
never had, you must
be willing to do
something you've
never done before."
– Thomas Jefferson

This section is the last but not least. It takes us back to where we started: We are the mirror of our lives. It is said, "Look at your friends and you will find out who you are." As we are transforming, some of those friends no longer serve our highest good and leave our lives, while new ones enter. This is a normal cycle of life and happy people will always hang out with happy people and *vice versa*.

Thomas Jefferson said: "If you want something you've never had, you must be willing to do something you've never done before. " This is what this 7-module guide is all about. It will enable you to open your mind to new horizons and help you change your behavior so you can have the "good health. good life." you all deserve.

To finish this section, I would like to use a fish metaphor. Fish don't know that there is this outside world. All they know is that there is an abundance of water where they swim. We, humans, are the same. We live in our realities and what we don't know is what we don't know. But you can start knowing with Module 1!

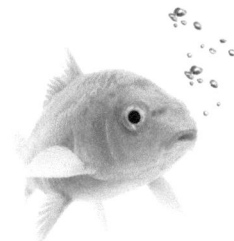

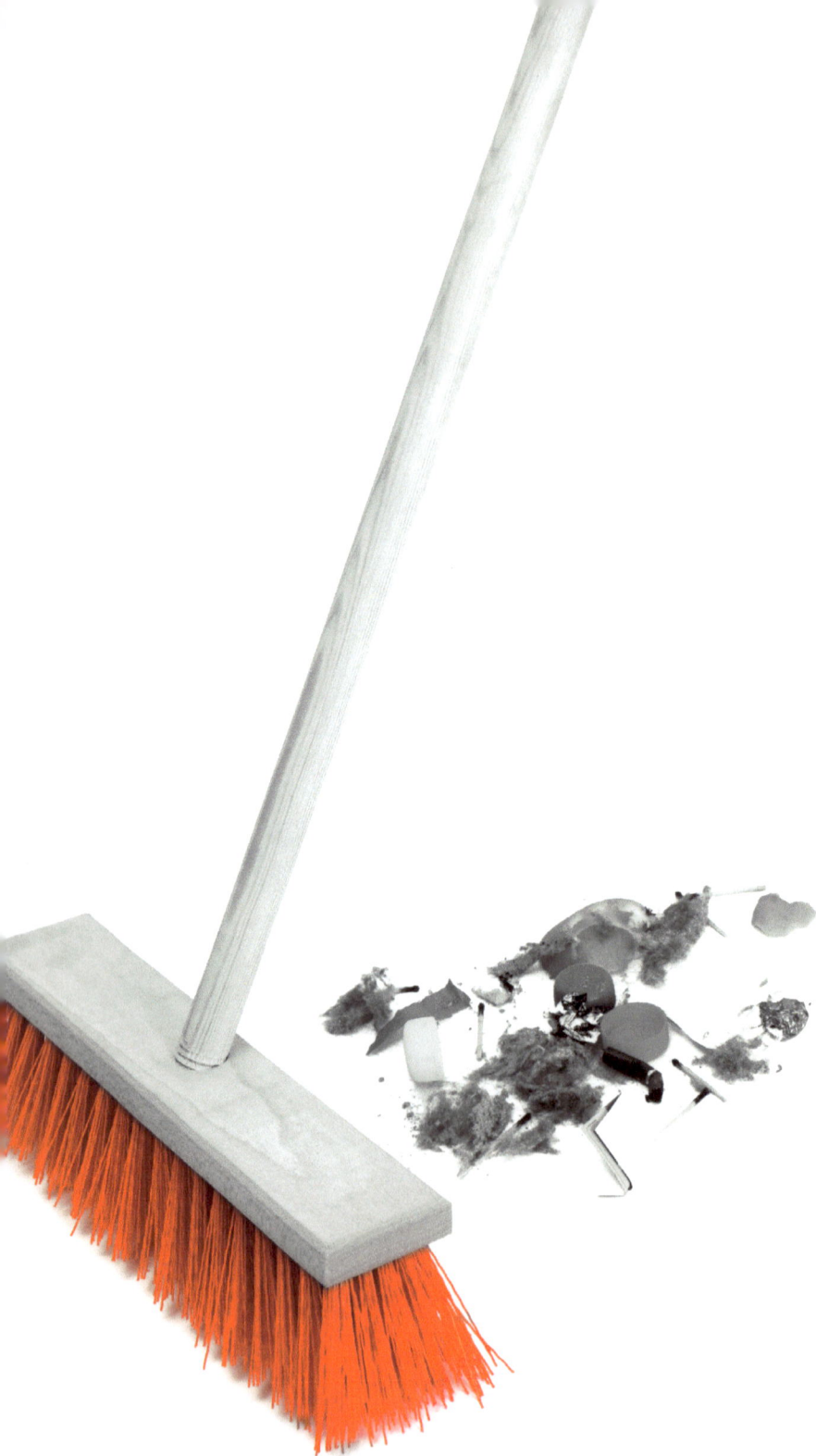

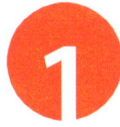

GOOD MIND: LET GO OF THE PAST

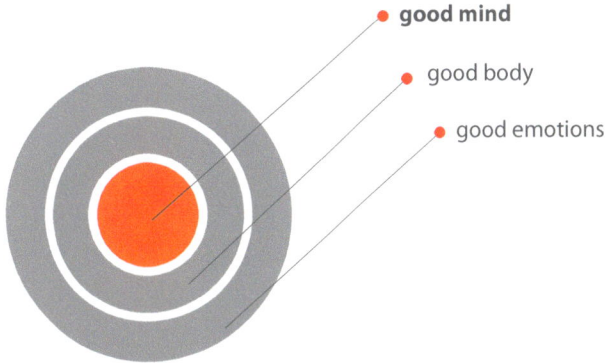

- **good mind**
- good body
- good emotions

Let go of the PAST	Be Positive. Be PRESENT	Manifest Your FUTURE
Understand and clear limiting beliefs and blocks that hold you back (a) consciously (b) sub-consciously.	Live the life you want to have NOW.	Identify your passions and talents and manifest a clear vision for your life.

The truth will set you free.

Picture yourself on one of the most beautiful white sandy beaches over-looking the deep blue ocean. You are the excited, joyful surfer swimming out to the ocean, patiently waiting for that perfect wave to approach you. The wave that is right for you and for your skills. You have been training to have the skills to get on that surfboard when the time is right. You seize the perfect moment, and you move with the wave with grace and ease. The wave takes you to the most extraordinary heights, to the most beautiful experience, and all you can do is to trust, have faith and enjoy. This is exactly the formula for living.

The winning formula for life is to slow down, enjoy the moment and patiently wait to seize our perfect wave. Instead, we often keep paddling toward that wave and, by the time it reaches us, we are too tired to get on it. The wave passes, but there will be another one if we just wait patiently. But we don't, so we keep paddling and again miss it because we are exhausted or distracted by other things around us.

We need to quiet the noise in our head by being still and calm, allowing ourselves to be guided and not worry, but to trust that the perfect wave arrives and we are ready when we are ready. This doesn't mean that we just wait and do nothing. We all need to know what kind of life we would like to live. Then let's grow into the person we would like to be, and take action to go after what we want. Meanwhile, have faith and trust in the process of the universe that it brings us the right people and circumstances to make our dreams come true. Do not worry. Be not afraid. Be patient. And believe that what we want is happening at the perfect time. It may not happen as fast as we want, but it happens exactly at the time when we are ready. Have you noticed, it always makes sense when we look back at our lives, but never when we are in the situation?

Our mind is the source of all being. What we think becomes true for us. However, what we think depends on the experiences we have had and how those experiences have conditioned our values and beliefs. To understand the present, we need to understand the past; because that past has shaped our present. If we keep doing what we always have done, the future will mirror the present and the past.

In order to change our lives, we need to let go, reshape those past conditionings so the present can start changing and the future will look a lot different from today. We want to identify and clear limiting beliefs and blocks related to fear and anger in all areas of life. Only then can we truly transform our lives. Just to be clear, the type of fear we are talking about is a limiting belief that holds us back from success; i.e. , "There are too many candidates, so there's no point applying for that position" (low self-esteem, self-worth), or, "It is too difficult to move to another location, so let's just stay where we are" (fear of uncertainty, need for control). There is another type of fear that kicks in when we really need it, the survival mechanism; i.e., when being chased by a tiger; then we really should be afraid and run for our life. So how do we know what those limiting beliefs are and how do we clear them?

First, let's start knowing where we are in our PRESENT life. In what areas of life are we satisfied and in what areas are we dissatisfied? This exercise will start guiding us to the blocks and limiting beliefs as they are related to areas where we are dissatisfied. Without this awareness, the process of change cannot begin. Do the following "The Life Map" exercise.

What does YOUR life look like?

Place a dot on the scale from 1 to 10 in each category to indicate your level of satisfaction within each area. Number 1 indicates dissatisfaction and 10 indicates satisfaction.

	1	2	3	4	5	6	7	8	9	10
CAREER – work/business										
FINANCES – savings/investments/security										
HEALTH – health/well-being										
PHYSICAL ACTIVITY – fitness/strength/energy										
LOVE – romantic partner/togetherness										
RELATIONSHIPS – friendships/peers/social life										
FAMILY – home environment										
JOY – hobbies/fun/entertainment										
INTELLECTUAL – learning/personal growth										
SPIRITUALITY – inner self-development										

Identify imbalances.

Realization of where you are is the first step. Congratulations! Most of you doing this exercise probably are thinking about your life for the first time in a long while.

Now you know where you are in life and it is time to discover how to close some of those gaps that you have identified.

1. Ask yourself why you have those gaps and imbalances in your life. The answer to this question will help you start identifying blocks, fears and limiting beliefs.

2. What can you begin doing differently NOW, 1 month, 3 months, 6 months from now to start bringing more joy and satisfaction into your life? The answers to this question will be quick wins in your life. Take little actions which will eventually turn into habits and change your life. We are all here to live an enjoyable, pleasant, amazing life. So don't wait another day to start bringing more joy into yours. Joy attracts more joy, love attracts more love – mirror the life you want to have.

This exercise works magically for most people. It gives you the time to reflect, to "stop and think" about your health, life and well-being. It makes you aware of all the good and not-so-good in your life so you can start making positive changes to enhance your health and your life.

Now let us move into the really interesting part, the PAST, the 90% of our brain, the subconscious mind. For most of us, this is a real mystery. The subconscious mind holds all the experiences since we were born and it also carries generational patterns. It records everything.

To best explain this: If your ancestors were starving, it is likely you are facing some challenges with weight and food because your body is trying to hold onto the weight in case of famine.

We all know that childhood and the teenage years form our values and beliefs. As children, we are open and vulnerable and whatever happens in childhood affects us for life. For example, some of us have had a situation when we were the last ones to be picked for the baseball team by our classmates because, perhaps, we were not the top performers athletically or were carrying a few extra pounds. At that point, we probably made a decision that, "From now on, I will strive academically and do everything it takes to succeed. I will show them who I am!" Thus, throughout our life, we are competing, striving to succeed academically and professionally to compensate for being slighted way back when. This may not be all bad, because it has made us very competitive and successful. But has it come at the expense of our happiness? Are we proving something to others or are we doing it because we are enjoying it?

Another example: When, as a 3-year-old, we were jumping around being happy, singing and laughing, perhaps someone found it annoying and we were reprimanded. From that moment on, we guard our feelings, our joy, our love, our singing, because we don't want to get hurt again.

We all have different stories and that's what makes us so unique. However, it is often difficult to remember those occasions because our bodies' natural defense mechanism blocks those negative events from coming into our conscious mind, but they are still sitting there somewhere in the subconscious mind, guiding our every move.

The good news is, once we identify those occasions when we are adults and realize how those occasions have shaped our belief and value system, we can forgive and release them.

According to Jacqueline Sidman, PhD, president of The Sidman Institute in Irvine, Calif., an internationally recognized expert in her field of freeing the subconscious mind, the most effective method is hypnotherapy (in this type of hypnotherapy, the patient remains conscious). As she says, we need to identify blocks where our defense mechanism kicks in because those are the limiting beliefs that hold us back. Your body is telling you, "Danger! Stop!"

"In hypnotherapy," says Sidman, "we go to the source of the defense and break through all the barriers." We want to release those early emotions and perceptions, often based on lies. When we face those lies now as adults, we can release all the negativity. We want to find out what happened consciously and that we are safe now and that will set us free. "Everybody needs it and everybody can benefit from it.," she concludes.

There are several techniques to clear limiting beliefs, the so-called blocks that hold us back. At the core of all those techniques is deep meditation, spirituality and prayer.

However, the first and the easiest step of clearing blocks is to start FACING the blocks, the key fears and insecurities in your life. There is a reason why they say go skydiving when you are frightened of heights. Sometimes, just addressing your fears will help you overcome them. Let go of the old, so the new can come in!

PRACTICAL TOOL 1-2: Block Identification PART 1

ANGER	•	I am angry at -
FEAR	•	I am afraid of -
GUILT	•	I feel guilty because -
WORRY	•	I am worried by -
UNFORGIVENESS	•	I haven't forgiven -
RESENTMENT	•	I resent -
HEARTBREAK	•	My heart is heavy because -
GRIEF	•	I feel grief because -
PRESSURE	•	I am so pressured by -
EXHAUSTION	•	I am exhausted because -
ANXIETY	•	I am anxious because -
STRESS	•	I am stressed because -
SHAME	•	I am ashamed of -
UNHAPPINESS	•	I am unhappy because -

Please note, this section may bring out some unexpected sensations because the purpose of the exercise is to help you remember why you are feeling the negative emotions that you are feeling. When you do experience emotions, you have started a healing process and it's the beginning of letting go. Realize that those situations were there for a reason, but they no longer serve any purpose, so it's time to let them go.

PRACTICAL TOOL 1-2: Block Identification PART 2

Once you have identified the blocks:

• Close your eyes

• Breathe deeply in and out

• Imagine a white bright light coming over you

• Ask the higher power to release those experiences for good

• Forgive!

• Thank the universe for taking care of them and bringing you all the love and joy

When you complete the exercise, you probably will feel lighter. Some of you may see physical pain disappearing as well. For example, when I did the release exercise, my lower back pain vanished. The hypnotherapy is even more effective. Some people have been healed of infertility and other conditions that are pretty hard to cure. Our emotional state is inherently linked to our physical body so, once we release the emotional pain, the physical pain disappears as well. This is exactly how Reiki, energy healing, works – by rebalancing the energy/the emotional body, the physical body gets healed as well.

Now let's be clear, we do not need to delete all of our past. But in order to manifest your dream life, both the subconscious and conscious mind need to be aligned. For example, if your belief system (your subconscious mind) believes in lack of abundance – "I can never be rich doing what I love" – then your conscious affirmations around the abundance – "Money comes easily to me" – will not materialize.

The subconscious mind knows when you are lying. The easiest way to change your subconscious is to change your WORDS. "What I say is who I become." The subconscious is your friend trying to listen to every command you make. Every word and thought is recorded in the subconscious; with enough repetition, it accepts them as commands. Positive life-enhancing words correspond strikingly fast. Successful prosperous words will open up channels for income. Words are manifesting a connection with the law of our being. The reason the subconscious mind is so important is because your life is mirroring your subconscious.

The last part of Letting Go of the Past is to **Detoxify Your Life – create space for the life you want to live.** The most rejuvenating experience of my life was to pack up my Wall St. apartment, give away most of what was left there, and leave my stressful corporate career. I felt like a boulder was lifted off my shoulders.

Stuff that has been sitting around for years means holding on to the past. It keeps you in the past. When you give it away, you let go and make space for the new. Only then can the universe start bringing you new things, new circumstances and new people, because you have made space for the new to come in.

Identify what things, foods, activities, situations and people no longer serve your highest good and let them go so the new can come in:

PRACTICAL TOOL 1-3: Detoxify Your Health and Your Life		
DETOXIFY YOUR **HOME**	•	Is your home representing you and who you are?
	•	Do you feel comfortable in your home?
	•	What could you change to make it more comfortable?
DETOXIFY YOUR **WARDROBE**	•	What has been sitting around for too long or is no longer you?
	•	Ask yourself, "Why do I still hold onto those things?"
DETOXIFY YOUR **REFRIGERATOR**	•	Is everything in your refrigerator that nourishes your body good for you (nutritious, healthy)?
	•	If not, why do you have it?
DETOXIFY YOUR **RELATIONSHIPS**	•	What could you stop doing to make your relationships with family and friends better?
	•	Are there people in your life who might be bad influence?
DETOXIFY YOUR **LIFE**	•	What are the activities that you could stop doing because those activities no longer serve your highest good?

To summarize, in this section of "LETTING GO OF THE PAST," we have accomplished a lot:

1. We have figured out **The Life Map** – how satisfied we are in important areas of our lives. We have identified actions and quick wins to start making small changes now.

2. We also have completed **Block Identification** where we identified, addressed and released fear and anger that have held us back.

3. We have started to **Detoxify Our Lives** by scanning for clutter, things and activities that are no longer good for us. We have learned to let go of the old so the new can come in.

As they say, "The truth will set you free."

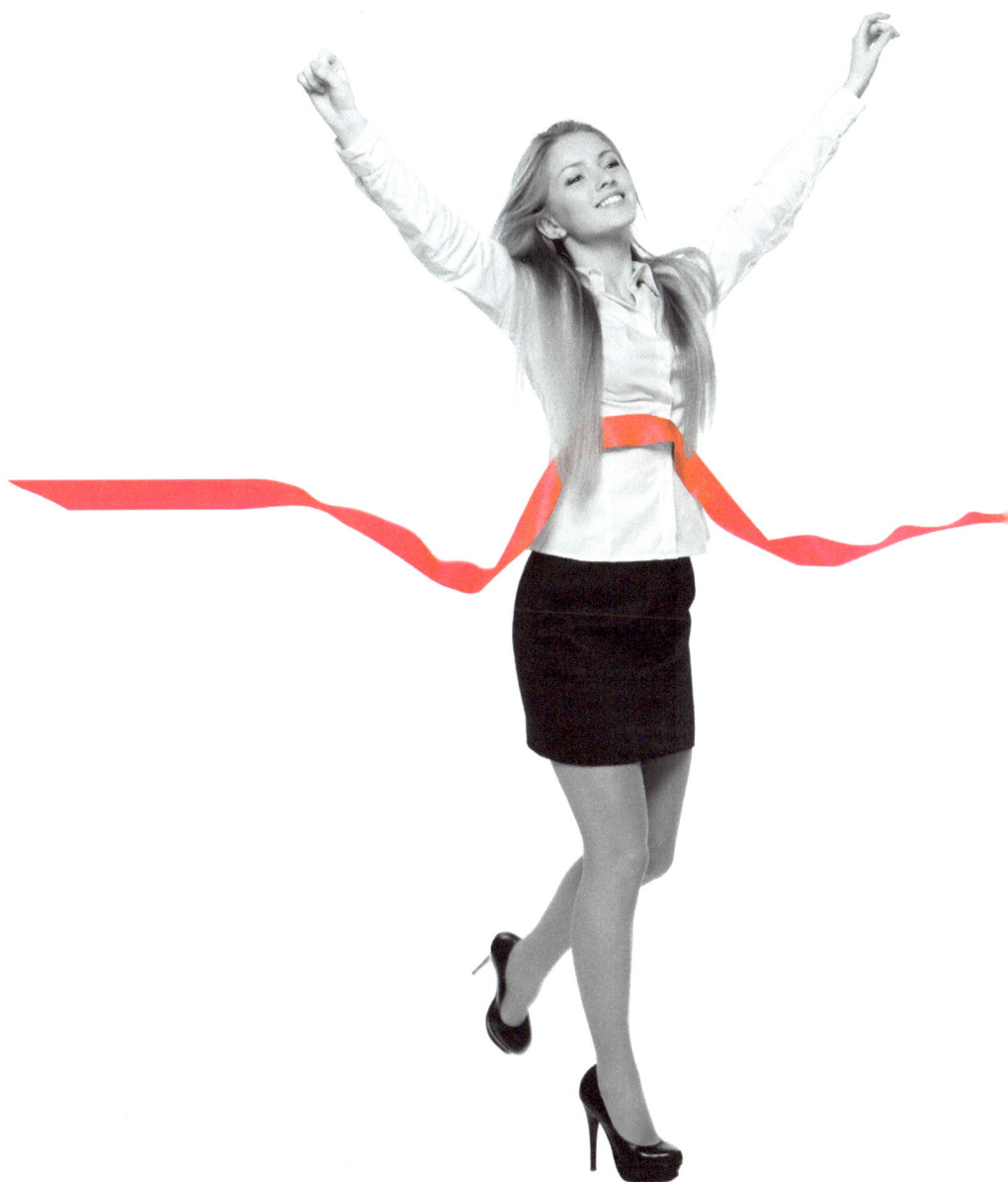

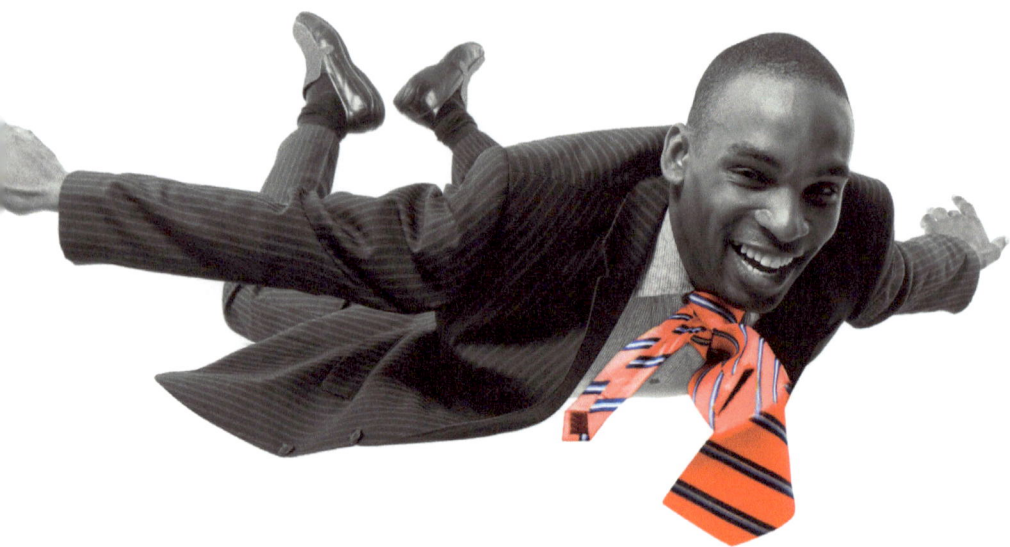

module

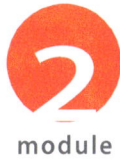

GOOD MIND: BE POSITIVE. BE PRESENT.

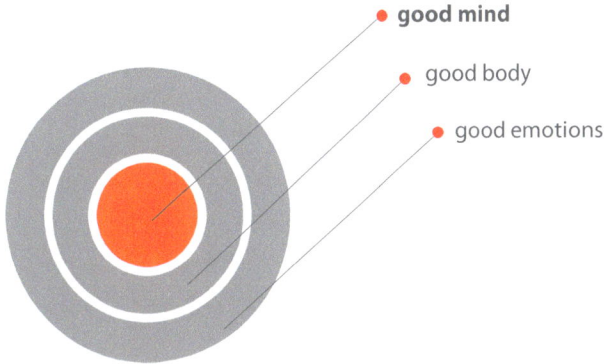

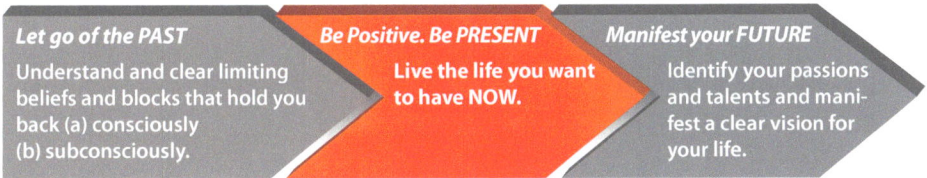

- **good mind**
- good body
- good emotions

Let go of the PAST	Be Positive. Be PRESENT	Manifest your FUTURE
Understand and clear limiting beliefs and blocks that hold you back (a) consciously (b) subconsciously.	Live the life you want to have NOW.	Identify your passions and talents and manifest a clear vision for your life.

Live the life you want to have NOW.

We have all heard of "be positive," "think positively" and then your life will magically turn into a happy place. How does it really work? It can't be that simple. Well, it actually is.

You now may be thinking, "When I get that new job, I will be content." or, "I wish I could meet my soul mate and then I'd be happy." or, "When the kids are off to college, we will start traveling and enjoying our lives." or, "If I could only have children, then all my dreams will have come true." The truth is, the list goes on forever and when you actually get those things, it may not turn out to be that perfect. How many times have you gotten that new job and it ends up being worse than the previous one? How many times have you met your soul mate and, suddenly, there are more problems in your life? Once you become a parent, how often do you just wish for peace and quiet?

The point is, this is a conditional type of happiness, where the target keeps moving away every time we get what we thought we wanted. So you might as well enjoy your life now because whatever you think you want is not going to bring you that fulfillment anyway. The lesson we need to learn in this life is to see the beauty around us every day, every moment, because that is all that is granted to us.

The BE-DO-HAVE model, which some say was first introduced by L. Ron Hubbard in his book, "Conditions of Existence," is LIVE the life you WANT to have NOW. Be happy now. Don't push it into the future. BE the career you want to HAVE now. DO the things you want to have now in order to have the life you want. In other words, "Based on what I want to be, I do the things I need to do, and the result is that I have what I want. "The assumption here is that we know what we want.

Yet, most of the time, we don't really know what we want because we have not had the time to think about it. We have always done the same thing. It's comfortable to be doing the same thing. I used to change jobs and companies, thinking my life will change if I get a new job in a new company, in a new city, in a new country. Guess what? Most of the time, nothing changed, or it got worse. Changing the label does not change the essence of it. We will dedicate Module 3 to identifying our passions and talents, and manifesting a clear vision, so stay tuned until then.

How can we shift our minds so we will not worry about the past or the future, but will really live and enjoy the NOW? There are a couple of practical tools that have helped me a lot and I am happy to share them with you. It all comes back to calming the noise in our MINDS, and slowing down. Because, if we don't slow down, we don't listen and that's when it is easy to make mistakes and rush into things we regret later. When we listen to our inner guidance, we will always make the right decision. The reason we need to be calm is because calm energy is positive energy that vibrates on the higher level, making it easier to manifest all our desires, wishes and dreams.

As you have probably heard, most successful people meditate. They may have not talked about it in the past, but now it is no longer a thing that only the yogis do. We often rush through our days, making us anxious and stressed. Meditation helps to calm our mind and slow us down. It is proven that 10 minutes of meditation a day can really change your life for good.

PRACTICAL TOOL 2-1: 10-minute Life-Changing Meditation Practice

• Set the timer for 10 minutes.

• Sit in a comfortable position or just lay down in bed; whatever works for you.

• Close your eyes and breathe in and out deeply.

• Relax your mind and body – face, neck, arms, legs, shoulders, back.

• In your mind, be grateful for what you have in your life. Just think for what you are grateful.

• Ask a specific question that has been on your mind or for the guidance you seek.

• Quiet your mind – try not to think about anything. Just listen to what comes up. This is the hardest part! Our mind wants to think, analyze, plan, wonder, etc. When thoughts come up, just let them go and be in a place of SERENITY.

This meditation exercise will help make you calmer, healthier and happier. It brings clarity and gets you more in touch with your inner guidance. For every person, the message and guidance is different. So pay attention and have a journal handy to write down ideas, thoughts, how your body feels, the messages you are getting.

If there is one single, most useful daily practice that will change your life for good, then it is MEDITATION!

One consistent thing between all living things is breathing. When we are balanced, our breathing is calm and relaxed. When we are stressed or anxious, our breathing will get more rapid and our blood pressure increases. In order to calm the stress and anxiety, we need to calm the breathing.

According to Dr. Andrew Weil, physician, naturopath, a teacher and writer on holistic health, founder, professor and director of the Arizona Center for Integrative Medicine at the University of Arizona, there is this 1½-minute breathing exercise that works wonders on stress and anxiety. Every time you feel stressed out, irritated, anxious or just need a good night's sleep, use this exercise.

PRACTICAL TOOL 2-2: 4/7/8 Stress-Relief Breathing in 1½ minutes

- Close your eyes

- Breathe IN, counting from 1 to 4

- HOLD your breath, counting from 1 to 7

- EXHALE, counting from 1 to 8

- Repeat this 4/7/8 breathing cycle 4 times

Do this 2 times a day whenever you feel anxious or stressed out.

By the way, my dad does this breathing exercise every night before he goes to bed and he sleeps like a baby and his blood pressure is under control.

As you have probably noticed, the NOW is directly correlated with breathing. Both (1) the Meditation and (2) the 1½-minute breathing exercise will help you calm your nervous system and calm you, too. Clarity only comes through stillness. Similarly, you will only see the bottom of the ocean when it is calm, not when it is unsettled. However, I understand how hard it is to be still when the world around you is stormy. Just remember, a calm vibration is a high vibration.

While the last two exercises help us get into the NOW, and make us more calm so we can start seeing clearly, the last exercise in this section will help us become more POSITIVE.

First, let's understand why we need to be positive.

Your thoughts are mainly what drive you on a physical level. It is your mind that tells you what to do, what you should learn and how you should act or react. With every thought, there is a reaction. This response can either energize you or decrease your life force. According to the laws of resonance, when negative thoughts are radiated to the environment, all thoughts on that morphogenetic field will be attracted. The negativity becomes stronger and happens more often. That's why people who have problems always seem to have problems. Similarly, people who are happy always seem to be happy. Like attracts like!

The truth is, life is not always smooth sailing. Things do come up that need to be addressed and could be quite upsetting. How you choose to see the world, your reaction, determines your success or failure. Even when situations come up that are not so positive, try to see good in those situations as well. What's the lesson you are meant to be learning? Why are you getting that lesson? Is the situation pushing you in a different direction? Try to look at those situations as your life path's correction tools. One of my mantras is to "Live life as if everything is rigged in your favor," a quote by 13th-century Persian poet Rumi, a theologian and Sufi mystic whose poems have been translated into many languages, including English.

Understand that being able to experience feelings is a blessing. We live in the world of polarities, i.e, hot & cold, good & evil, soft & hard, light & dark, short & long, masculine & feminine, etc. The polar opposites enable us to experience feelings. Without polarity, we would not be able to feel anything.

Alright, enough of philosophy; let's get practical. The easiest way to become more positive is to do more things that we like, enjoy and love. Take the time to think about what you like, what you do not like and what you really want. This exercise will reveal your energetic field and what you attract into your life. Just thinking about what you like and what you want will start opening up new possibilities.

PRACTICAL TOOL 2-3: Positivity Assessment		
What do I like in my life?	What do I not like in my life?	What do I really want?

Our goal is to start doing more of the things we like and less of the things we don't like, or find a way to make the not-so-likable things more enjoyable. We need to remove the interferences.

To summarize: We have accomplished a lot in this section of "BE POSITIVE. BE PRESENT."

1. We have learned how to become more PRESENT by calming our minds so we can start listening and seeing what's good for us. There are two transformational practical tools: The 10-minute Meditation and Dr. Weil's 1½-minute breathing exercise that will greatly help you polish that skill.

2. We have learned the importance of POSITIVITY and how like attracts like. So let's work on our mind shift and how to see our lives in a more positive, magical way by bringing more joy into our lives.

Keep your thoughts positive
because your thoughts
become your WORDS.
Keep your words positive
because your words
become your BEHAVIOR.
Keep your behavior positive
because your behavior
becomes your HABITS.
Keep your habits positive
because your habits
become your VALUES.
Keep your values positive
because your values
become your DESTINY.

– Mahatma Gandhi

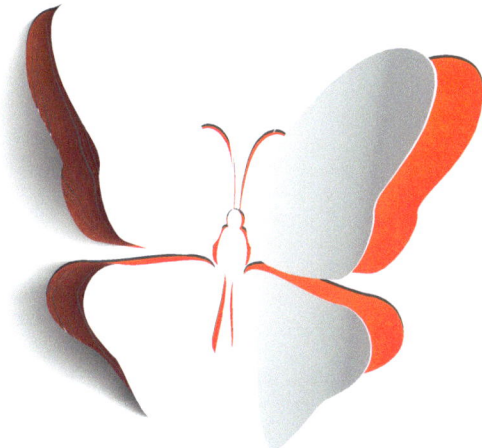

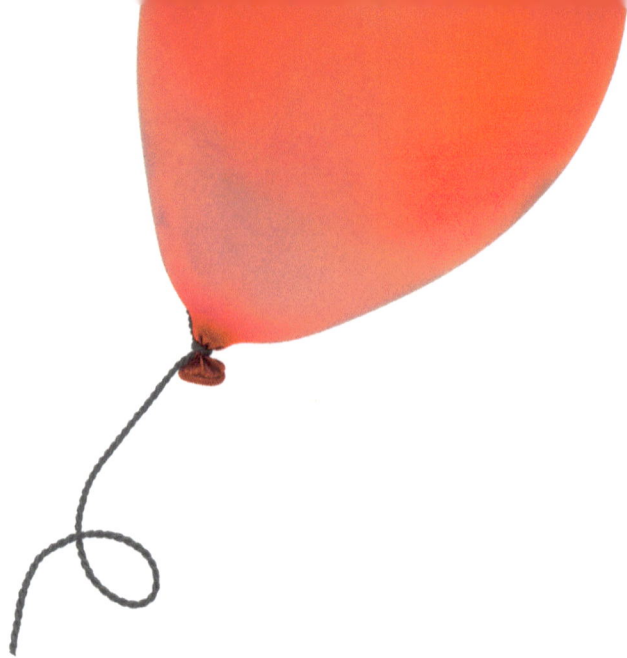
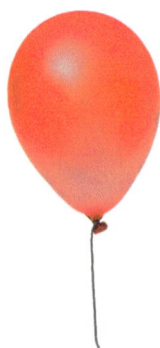
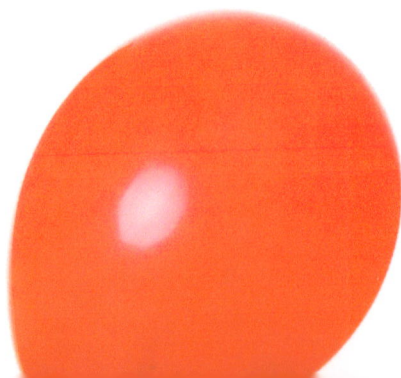

GOOD MIND: MANIFEST YOUR FUTURE.

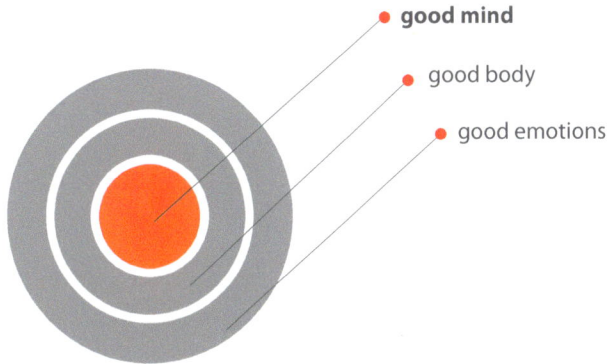

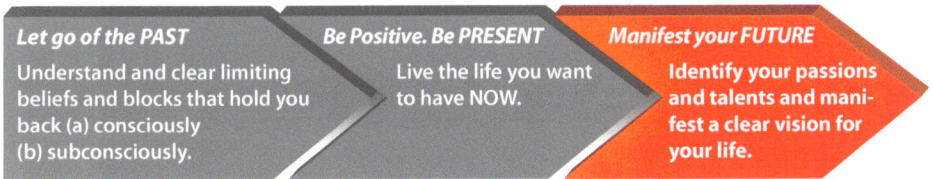

- **good mind**
- good body
- good emotions

Let go of the PAST

Understand and clear limiting beliefs and blocks that hold you back (a) consciously (b) subconsciously.

Be Positive. Be PRESENT

Live the life you want to have NOW.

Manifest your FUTURE

Identify your passions and talents and manifest a clear vision for your life.

Live from the highest possible version of You.

Our life is a journey of self-discovery. On our paths, we need to dive deep within ourselves, figuring out our most unique and powerful gifts and use them to enrich our lives as well as the lives of others.

What we think about and on what we focus, we tend to attract to us and create in our lives. Knowing this, we should really be clear about who we are and what we want in life, because our thoughts and actions will start guiding us there, and have guided us to where we are today.

Surprisingly, most people are not being true to themselves because they are not clear about who they are and what they want, or they think they do and then they get it and realize they have been on the wrong path all their life. We often spend more time planning for our job objectives and strategies than thinking about our own lives. I used to be one of those people. I don't think I ever took the time to think about what my talents are, what I really enjoy, at what I am really good, and what comes naturally and easily to me. I always followed a comfortable, easy path of changing companies and progressing in my career and doing things I thought successful people should do, but I didn't really live a life I enjoyed. When I started thinking about my life , who I am, what I want, what I like, my life started shifting in the right direction – one step at a time. It didn't happen overnight, but it was all worth the wait.

The first exercise I did was create a list of my passions and my talents. I even asked my closest friends to tell me at what I am really proficient. Often those talents come so easily and naturally to us that it is easy to ignore them, or we just take them for granted.

PRACTICAL TOOL 3-1: Who Am I?	
What are my PASSIONS?	**What are my TALENTS?**

Once I was done with the exercise, the surprising fact was that all my talents listed were actually related to my work experience, because that's the face I always have shown to the world. Basically, even my closest friends really didn't know me, didn't know my passions, or what I truly love and enjoy! I had been hiding all those years behind labels and credentials, showing the side of me I thought the world wants to see rather than living from the highest possible version of me.

My life began changing when I created a VISION BOARD for my life, and a ROADMAP. I cut out photos and words from different magazines and started creating a collage notebook of the life I wanted to have and wrote down specific goals with time-frames. In other words, I started telling the universe WHAT I want.

PRACTICAL TOOL 3-2: My Life's Vision Board

• **Take a notebook and start adding photos and words from different magazines that resonate with you and best describe the life you want. You will end up with a beautiful PHOTO ALBUM/COLLAGE.**

PRACTICAL TOOL 3-3: My Life's Roadmap

• **Write down GOALS you want to achieve by the end of: 1 month, 3 months, 6 months, 1 year, 2 years, 3 years, 5 years, 10 years, 15 years, 20 years, 25 years, etc.** Capture everything you want to have, but write it as though you already have it. This will condition the brain to think that you do already have it.

Note: Don't over-specify the list. Articulate WHAT you want but not HOW you are going to get it. Always manifest in the NOW like you already have it (no "will" or "want").

MY GOALS

Month 1	Month 3

Month 6	Year 1

Year 2	Year 3

Year 5	Year 10

The last exercise in "MANIFEST YOUR FUTURE" is writing down AFFIRMATIONS – thanking the universe as though you already have everything you want. For example, "Thank you, universe, for making me beautiful inside and out and letting my greatness shine." or, "Thank you, universe, for making me a millionaire."

PRACTICAL TOOL 3-4: My Affirmations

"Thank you, universe, for ...

Related to the BE-DO-HAVE model, it is important to start witnessing what you want: visualize, imagine, experience and feel it. Affirmations help us strengthen our belief system that what we want, we already have.

Yes, this is all very simple, but all good things in life are simple. Just taking the time to think about your life and what you want is a major step in the right direction.

Once the vision, roadmap and affirmations have been completed, let's understand **How to Manifest Your Ideal Life.** The most important part of manifesting your future is to be POSITIVE, because a positive mind has a higher vibration. The higher the vibration, the more likely you will manifest. Everything in life is energy and similar energy attracts similar energy. Things that have higher vibration resonate at the higher, at the positive level, and things with lower vibration operate at the lower, negative level. So, back to like attracts like. Our goal is to operate at the higher vibration because that's the only way we can attract more positivity into our lives – love, joy, peace and happiness.

In addition to being positive, we also need to TAKE ACTION. Buy that lottery ticket, start a company or do something that enables things in your life to start happening, manifesting!

Simple ways to increase your energy vibration and manifest:

• **"What you resist, persists"** • The universe doesn't know the difference between positive and negative. Whatever you hate, you are also empowering and drawing into your life. Remove the interferences, the things you don't like.

• **Visualize and feel the abundance in your life** • Have positive emotions and feelings because like attracts like and that energy will bring circumstances into your life where you can feel that way. In other words, shift out of frustration if you don't want to have more of that feeling.

• **Align with your purpose** • Be who you really are, showing all your talents and gifts.

• **Release attachment to result** • Let go and trust that it happens. Take a leap of faith!

• **Live fully in the moment** • The more you are happy with what you have right now, the more likely you are getting what you are manifesting.

• **Move beyond fear** • Fear and anger shut down manifestation.

• **Make peace with your past** • Your beliefs must be in line with your goals; heal beliefs inside that limit you.

• **Detoxify your life** • Remove all things and people you don't need anymore; they hold you back.

• **Affirmations & action** • "I always do what needs to be done."

• **Gratitude list** • Make a list of everything for which you are grateful. This helps you focus on the abundance rather than the lack of it.

• **Meditate/breathing** • We do this to calm our energy and, as stated, calm vibration is higher vibration. Get out of the thinking mode and get into your heart.

• **Be active** • Exercise releases dopamine, the pleasure hormone. The happier we feel, the higher the vibration.

• **Acts of kindness** • Volunteering, donating and giving is a great way to show the universe your abundance. Abundance is a high vibration.

• **Be in nature** • Life is amazing and truly beautiful from sunrise to sunset, from budding flowers to singing birds. Enjoy it! Love and joy are high vibration.

To summarize: Anything on which we focus will materialize in our lives. In order to have the life we want, we need to live from the highest possible version of us. When we find that inner balance, the outside world takes care of itself because we are the mirrors of our lives. Completing the Practical Tool: "Who Am I?" is the beginning of a self-discovery journey.

Once we know who we are and stay true to ourselves, we can start creating our Life's Vision and start Manifesting. Three "My Ideal Life" practical tools will put you on the track of making all your dreams come true: (1) My Vision Board (2) My Roadmap (3) My Affirmations.

Finally, as we figure out what we want, we need to start living it, taking action! Words define who we are and what we want. Because our thoughts lead to words, words lead to action. So choose your words carefully and make sure they are aligned with your vision, what you want in your life. If you don't like where you are today, change your thoughts, your words, your actions and create a new reality. Begin seeing things in a new way: If everything seemed gloomy before, start seeing how much beauty is around you and how much you have for which to be grateful, even if it is little things. Your perspective is your reality, so when your perspectives change, your reality will change as well.

> Eliminate words that
> represent what you
> don't want.
> If you don't want it,
> don't say it!

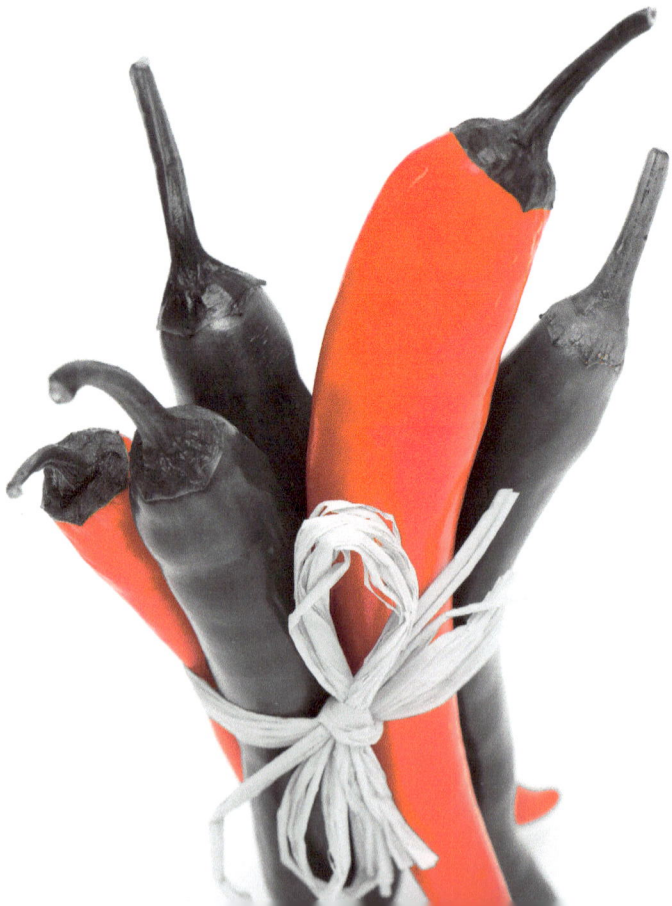

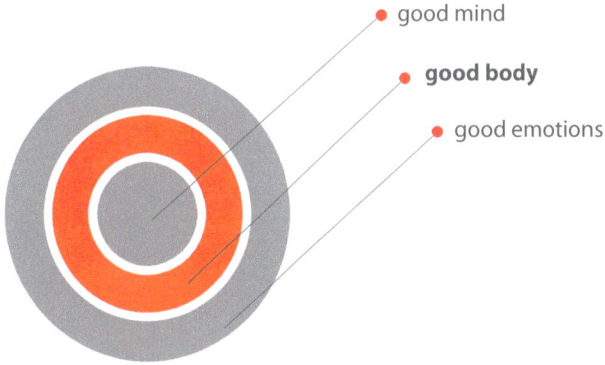

4

module

GOOD BODY: YOU ARE WHAT YOU EAT

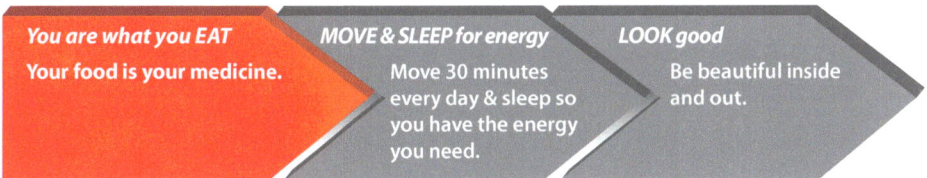

- good mind
- **good body**
- good emotions

| **You are what you EAT**
Your food is your medicine. | **MOVE & SLEEP for energy**
Move 30 minutes every day & sleep so you have the energy you need. | **LOOK good**
Be beautiful inside and out. |

Listen to your body!

Our bodies are the most automated, intelligent factories known to mankind. They know exactly what we need, and when and if something is missing. The body even is equipped to heal itself. All we need to do is listen to our body and take a good care of it. When we start feeling hungry, it is time to eat. When we feel full, it is time to stop eating. When we feel thirsty, it is time to hydrate ourselves. When we feel tired, it is time to rest. When we feel pain, it is time to slow down and recover. When we feel full of energy, it is time to push ourselves to the next level.

Food is the fuel of life. Good fuel will make us go further and faster, and bad fuel is likely to cause problems. We need good food for energy in order to keep going; but most of us struggle with food. Somehow, food has turned into an enemy rather than a loving partner. How often do we think about food – what and when we should or should not eat, how many calories, how much fat, how much sugar, yo-yo dieting, and the list continues.

I remember how, as a busy professional, I spent a big chunk of my day thinking about food, eating and dieting because I was struggling to maintain my weight.

First, stress had a lot do with it because, when we are stressed, the stress hormone cortisol not only increases our appetite but it also slows our metabolism and promotes fat storage. Thus, managing stress is critical for achieving healthy weight and body.

Second, the food served in our office cafeteria was not the kind that offered nutrition for energy (I understand how managing costs is critical for any business). In other words, it was quite an effort to eat healthy. The vending machines made it even worse. I gained 10 pounds, felt sluggish and tired. Finally, I decided to take my health into my own hands and began bringing my own breakfast, lunch and snacks to the office. The pounds started to fly off. As I got healthier, I even had energy to work out a couple of times a week. However, I did spend extra time at home planning and preparing my food for the next day. Since we spend about 10 hours five days a week in the office, it is important to fuel ourselves properly; otherwise it is easy to get run-down and burn out.

Home-cooking actually may turn out to be one of the most relaxing activities you do a couple of evenings a week. I always cooked a proper meal on Sunday that I could bring to the office the next couple of days, and something easy and simple Wednesday evenings. The other days, it was just combining some high-quality ingredients like prosciutto with melon or raw almonds for snacks, or a soft-boiled egg or yogurt with berries for breakfast. Home-cooking is a lot of fun, especially if you can cook together with a friend or loved one. When you bring the leftovers to the office, you reminisce about all that fun and love. It's a great way to make your long office day more enjoyable.

As busy professional men and women, we have too many other things on our minds to be thinking about food all the time. What we need is a balanced approach that keeps us healthy, full of energy and productive while working hard. The keys to success are (1) our relationship with food, (2) the amount and quality of food we eat, and (3) managing stress.

What worked for me, and has worked for most people, is changing our relationship with food. Food is something to be enjoyed, not something that stirs up feelings of guilt and despair. We need to love the food, not deprive ourselves of it.

When you follow the guidance in this section, you will likely not be on a diet again but will change your relationship with food for good. Food is an integral part of our beautiful life and it is an element of our enjoyable daily living when we eat good food with friends and family.

But I do understand that we all have special relationships with food, often linked to our childhood, whether it was a scarcity of food or we had to eat everything on our plate even when we were not hungry. Those patterns govern our daily lives now and the only way to change it is to realize why we are eating the way we do, face it now as adults and release that limiting belief for good. Once that mind shift change takes place, we'll start seeing food very differently and the pounds will fall off, since our bodies are naturally programmed to reach that ideal weight that makes us feel most comfortable.

For example, when you were a child and experienced food shortages, you may be binge-eating now. Despite being full, you probably never will leave anything on the plate. This all comes from the memory of food being scarce and that you didn't know from where your next meal was coming. Now, as an adult, you realize what is driving this behavior and you can tell your body that there is plenty of food; no need to eat everything you see. Just recognizing this will help you start seeing food in a more positive way.

PRACTICAL TOOL 4-1: Childhood Eating Habits

Take a moment to recall your family's eating habits during your childhood. This will be very revealing and will help you go to the source of the problem, rather than alleviating symptoms by trying different diets.

- Did you have enough food?
- Did you eat real food or fast food?
- Did you drink water, tea or soda?

- Did you snack on chocolate bars and candy rather than eating an apple?
- Did you have to finish all the food on your plate?
- Did your mom cook at home or did you mostly eat pre-made, processed foods?
- Did you eat together as a family or did you eat on the go?
- Do you recall anything else that is directly related to your current eating behavior and how you view food?

Once you realize those childhood patterns that you still are practicing today, just understand why things were the way they were back then. Given that your circumstances have changed, let that past go. Then take action to consciously change those patterns.

- If there was scarcity of food, tell your body you have plenty of food now and it will never run out.
- If you were eating fast food or processed foods, change to real food.
- If you drank soda as a kid, start drinking tea and water instead.

In other words, begin taking different actions so your behavior patterns can start changing, and your body will thank you in a couple of months' time.
I understand this is not as easy as it sounds because, for example, sugar is addictive because it over-stimulates the reward centers of the brain, i.e. you get the "sugar high" for a moment. This is how sugar "takes over" the brain and makes us crave and eat more, leading to weight gain. So first try cutting back ; it's a great step in the right direction!

One of my enduring childhood memories is of my mother's fabulous cooking. She could make anything taste great and she instilled in me a deep appreciation for good food cooked well. She always used farm-fresh ingredients, and made everything from scratch. I am truly grateful to her for providing me and my family with all the home-cooking despite being a full-time working mom. I believe it has played a big part in my feeling so healthy as an adult. I love food and food loves me.

Healthy eating starts from changing your relationship with food and seeing it as something to be enjoyed while you're relaxed and happy, rather than emotional eating to comfort you and make you feel better when you are stressed out.

We tend to attract to us and create in our lives what we think about and on what we focus. A very effective approach for changing your negative eating habits to positive ones that transform your body and life is to say affirmations and practice visualization as discussed in Module 3.

PRACTICAL TOOL 4-2: Weight-Loss Affirmations

Create a list of affirmations and visualize how perfect you already look NOW, and think like you already HAVE what you want:

- "I am slim, fit and beautiful."
- "Weight loss comes easily to me. Pounds just fall off."
- "I listen to my body and nourish my body with foods that are good for me, energize me, and make me feel good."
- "I love my fit body."
- "I have an abundance of time to take care of my body."

By changing your thoughts and beliefs, you instantly can change your emotional state.

After all, food is one of our main life sources. It nourishes us, keeps us strong and healthy and lifts our energy levels. When you view food in this way, and eat real foods that are good for you, the weight will drop off and you will feel amazing. On the other hand, when you view food as the enemy, the reason you have put on those extra few pounds, you will remain stuck in that yo-yo dieting. The cycle of deprivation and prize takes over – the prize often being sugar that gives you that short-lived high, followed by a feeling of tiredness and, ultimately, guilt.

So how do we stop this cycle of yo-yo dieting and change our bodies for good?

First, we need to detoxify our bodies from all the toxins that are stored in the fat cells. When you are dieting, you may have noticed that you feel tired, lethargic and headachy. Your body quickly decides that it doesn't like feeling that way and starts holding on to fat in order to store toxins so you can start feeling better. So the yo-yo dieting continues. The key is to stick to real foods that are unprocessed and close to their natural state (all-natural, organic, grass-fed or wild). Then you lose weight easily and keep it off. Before beginning the detoxifying program, let's cover some basics.

What are real foods?

- They haven't changed much from their natural state. For example, a potato looks like a potato that was picked from the ground rather than chips that have been processed. Choose quality over quantity and price.
- They are "all-natural'" or "organic" and don't have preservatives that make them last for months or years. The real foods spoil quickly because they are natural.
- They don't have any artificial colorants, sweeteners or flavorings.
- They have not been treated with growth hormones, GMOs (genetically modified organisms) or other artificial enhancers, or pesticides.
- They don't include hydrogenated fats, i.e. trans fat.
- The ingredient list is very simple (maximum 5 ingredients) that you can recognize and pronounce.

Let's also understand the key "good health. good life." eating principles for reaching your ideal body weight:

• SUGAR MAKES YOU FAT • If you eat sugar every day, you are likely struggling to lose weight. Sugar also leaks vitamins from your body, and a body starved of vitamins is a hungry one. That's one of the reasons why overweight people are always hungry; they don't eat nutritious food and are malnourished. It also makes you tired and weakens your immune system. Simply said, you may be used to sweets, but if you don't change those taste buds to "not so sweet," nothing will change. Sugar converts to fat quicker than fat itself, because it raises your insulin levels, which causes fat storage. Studies show that 40% - 60% of the sugar you eat is converted straight to fat, depending if you are a slim or overweight person. *Tip: Replace your sugar with honey.*

My parents tried this and, amazingly, the first pot of honey was gone in three days but, after that, the next one remained on the table for weeks, if not months. My hypothesis is that honey has a lot of vitamins and minerals. And my parents probably were lacking a lot of those in their high sugar use and, once the vitamins and minerals were replaced, the cravings disappeared. *Tip: Fruit juice has a lot of sugar, so eat real fruit instead, but no more than two a day.*

• CUT THE CRAPS • This would include

Refined sugar in cakes, cookies, sweets, "diet" foods and drinks, artificial sweeteners, and soda. *Tip: At least 70% pure or raw cocoa dark chocolate once in a while is OK!*

Alcohol that is full of sugar and, as a result, makes you fat around the middle. *Tip: A glass of good quality (ideally organic) red wine packed with antioxidants is okay once in a while!*

Processed foods made of too many unknown ingredients, full of manmade preservatives and additives and often packed with sugar to make them look appe-tizing (and get you addicted to them). Try to stay away from bread, pasta, white rice, canned fruit, ready meals, most cereals and, of course, chips. *Tip: The less a food has been altered, the better it is for you.*

Caffeine – good in small doses (2 cups of coffee per day). More than that will affect your sleep, especially if you have had caffeine after 2 p.m. Too much caffeine puts stress on your system. *Tip: Drink green or black tea instead. They are great metabolic, immune system boosters; plus, they are known to be calming and relaxing (opposite to stress).*

• STRESS IS THE WORST TOXIN IN THE ENTIRE BODY • WORSE THAN SUGAR •
When you are stressed, the stress hormone cortisol not only increases your appetite, but it also slows your metabolism and promotes fat storage. So managing stress and balancing our energy levels is critical to achieving healthy weight and body. *Tip: Don't forget the 10-minute meditation and 1½-minute breathing exercises introduced in Module 2 to help make you calm and relaxed. Exercise is also a great way to fight stress.*

• GOOD FAT IS GOOD FOR YOU • The heart-friendly fats found in nuts, avocados and oily fish, and oils (extra virgin olive oil, coconut oil) are good for you and actually help you lose weight. They should be eaten every day because they encourage your body to burn fat around your middle, and to absorb vitamins and minerals more efficiently. Good fats also reduce sugar cravings, increase your energy levels and keep you full longer.

• DRINK PURE WATER THROUGHOUT THE DAY • Replace soda drinks with water or tea. Water helps the body to flush out toxins. Drink water when you are thirsty. *Tip: Warm water with lemon has been used historically for detoxifying and cleansing. Feel free to add lemon or cucumber slices or mint leaves into your water to make it taste amazing.*

• KEEP IT SIMPLE •
- Prepare foods simply and naturally.
- Never count calories.
- Choose a varied diet that does not involve the same foods over and over to ensure food intolerance does not develop.
- Try not to eat later than 7 p.m. This is to allow your body enough time to digest before you go to bed. Never overeat. Be 80% full.
- Good food tastes amazing. Enjoy every mouthful!

As stated at the beginning of this module, detoxifying your body from all the toxins is the very first step of starting to achieve "good health. good life." There are many ways to detoxify your body. Some prefer to go away to a detoxification retreat and have a guided program to cleanse the body, mind and spirit. Others are too busy and need a DIY version like the one I suggest below.

PRACTICAL TOOL 4-3: Detoxify Your Body – 7-Day Plan

The purpose of this detoxification program is to cleanse and repair all the major organs through nutrition and good habits that will set you up for a lifetime of good health. Please note, this plan does NOT involve fasting, as we all need our energy to be productive.

- Give up caffeine, alcohol and sugar for 7 days.
- Eat real foods, preferably "organic," "all-natural," "wild," "pure" and "unsweetened".
- Drink pure water throughout the day (don't forget the lemon!).
- Do a gentle exercise such as yoga, Pilates, tai chi or walking.
- Try to treat yourself to at least one massage and/or one Reiki session to get the toxins moving and exiting your body.
- Create meals from the following menu suggestions:

Breakfast Choose from:	Lunch Choose from:	Dinner (light and easily digestible – not raw) Choose from:
• Fresh fruit: apple, pear, orange, grapefruit, kiwi, peach, nectarine, tangerine, banana or pineapple (You can add or choose any of these.)	• Green leafy salad: watercress, shredded cabbage, arugula, spinach, cooked beets, tomatoes, parsley, boiled artichoke hearts, carrots, fennel, celery, cucumber, lettuce (You can add or choose any of these.)	• Cottage cheese on rye bread
• Fresh fruit (strawberries, raspberries or blueberries) with yogurt and chopped nuts (almonds or walnuts)	• For a dressing, squeeze lemon juice (1/3 of a lemon), 1 tablespoon extra virgin olive oil, sea salt, pepper	• Lightly boiled or steamed vegetables: broccoli, asparagus, green beans, artichokes, cauliflower, brussels sprouts, peas, squash, zucchini, sweet potatoes (your choice) with garlic, lemon, extra virgin olive oil, sea salt
• Fresh fruit with chopped nuts and muesli	• Have this either with fish, chicken, cottage cheese or beans or with avocado and 1 slice of good-quality bread (rye or sprouted wheat)	• Fresh vegetable soup with chopped herbs and barley
• Poached or soft-boiled egg with tomatoes or ½ avocado		
• Non-sweet cereal with almond or rice milk or organic milk		

This detoxification plan is truly good for you, your health and well-being. It involves a slow but deliberate change in what you eat and how you eat it. It will kick-start your body, your system for weight loss, and good food and nutrition for life. During the first few days of your detoxification, you may experience typical symptoms of lethargy, headache and irritability. This is because toxins are being released and need to be wiped off quickly and efficiently to minimize these effects and maximize the benefits. It is all worth it because, at the end, you will look healthier, your skin will get firmer, your hair will be shiny, you will have more energy, and your body will feel lighter. Some say they even look younger!

The detoxification process is dependent on having a ready source of antioxidants, phytonutrients, essential fats and B vitamins to make certain your organs have the fuel and the help they need to cleanse your body as quickly as possible. Supplements help ensure you get your daily requirements of micronutrients that may be missing from your diet. So it is important to start taking high-quality, purest EPA/DHA Omega 3 fish oil, multivitamins and probiotics supplements daily.

You are what you eat. Food can make you feel energized, slim, fit and young. It has the power to make your eyes brighter, your skin glow and your hair shine. But it can also make you feel bad if you eat the wrong type of food. It can make you feel fat, bloated, tired and guilty. So next time, when you are ready to enjoy your breakfast, lunch or dinner, think about how you would like to feel. Ultimately, it is your choice.

Listen to your body;
it knows when it is
hungry and when it
has had enough.

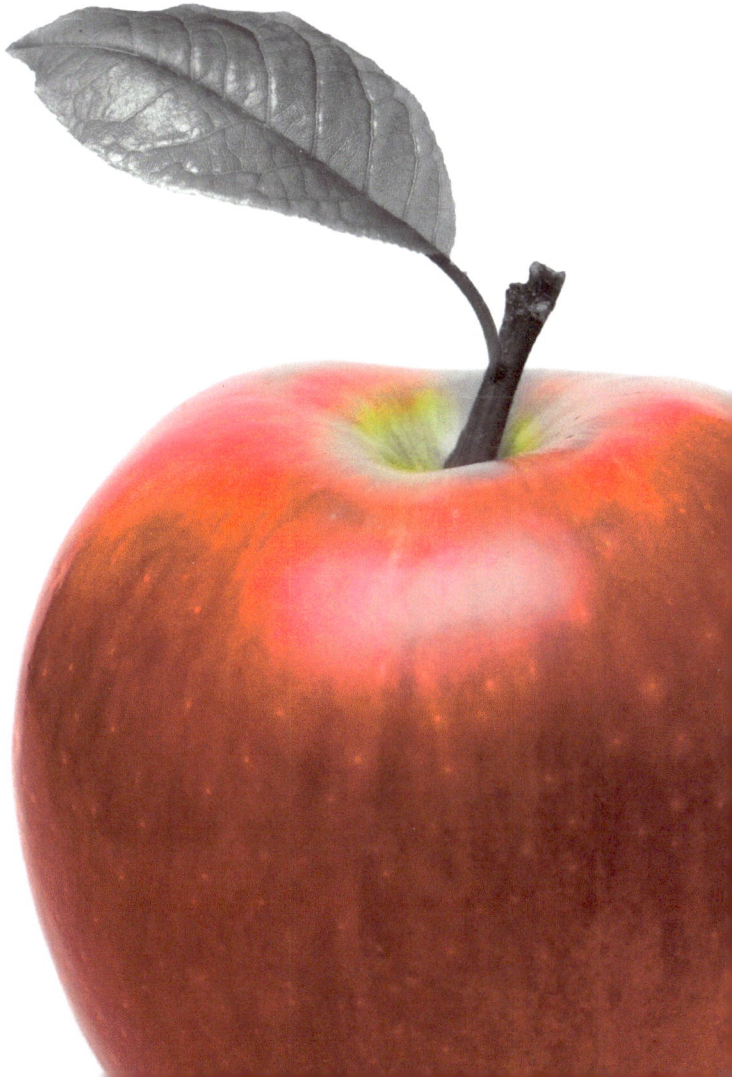

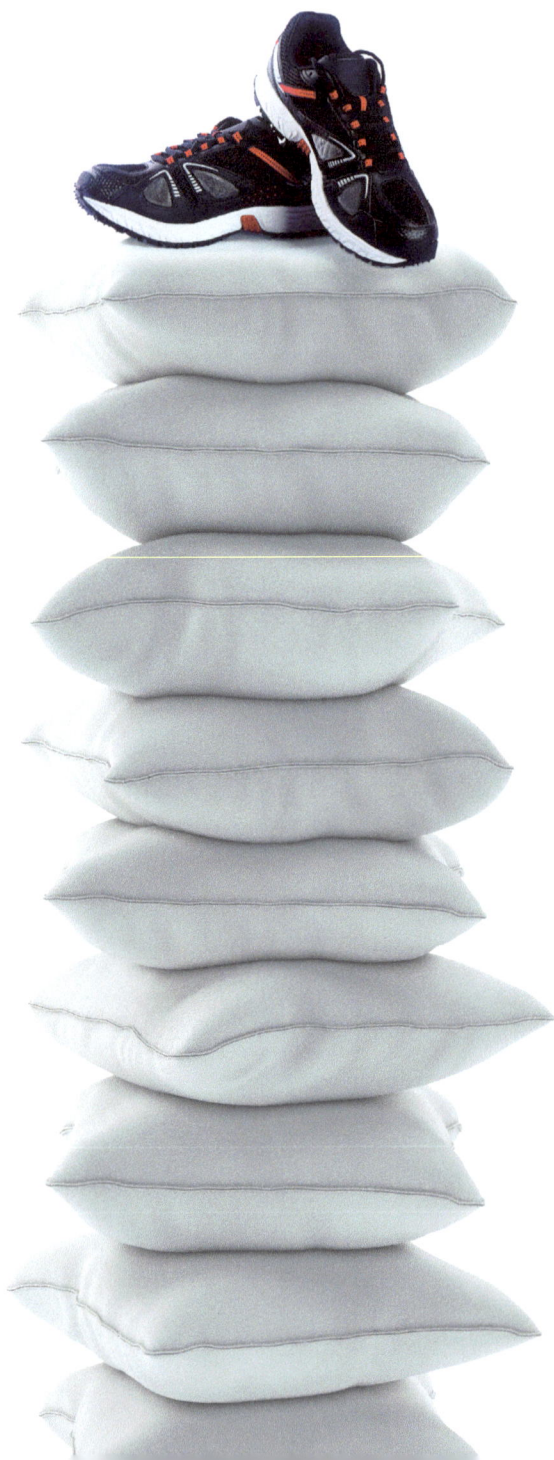

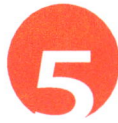

5

module

GOOD BODY:
MOVE & SLEEP FOR ENERGY

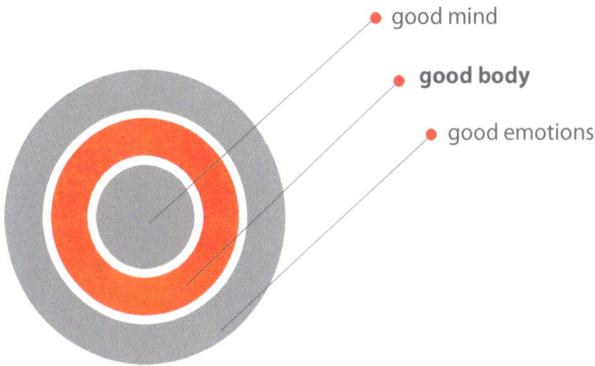

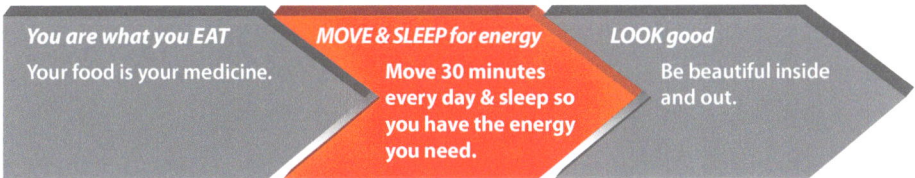

- good mind
- **good body**
- good emotions

You are what you EAT	*MOVE & SLEEP for energy*	*LOOK good*
Your food is your medicine.	**Move 30 minutes every day & sleep so you have the energy you need.**	Be beautiful inside and out.

It's all about energy balance.

Everything in this world is energy. Whatever you are vibrating, you attract. The more attention you pay to something, the more attention it pays to you. You cannot focus on sickness and attract health. Correct the imbalance between your current state and your desired state by interacting with greater energy sources that vibrate with your desired qualities: everything from your thoughts to the people with whom you hang out, to the foods you eat; everything with which your senses come in contact. Be conscious of the choices you make!

The way to maximize your own energy is to be balanced, to be comfortable in your own skin. When you are balanced inside, the outside world takes care of itself. The way to keep your energy balanced is to have a balanced state of mind, body and emotions. Basically, listen to your body and your body will tell you what it needs. In order to have the balanced energy, you need the integrative approach to well-being focusing on everything, from nutrition to stress management, along with exercise, physiology and sleep habits. And as the mind is connected to everything, if one of them is out of order, you will feel it.

True energy comes from a healthy digestive system. We covered everything about nutrition in Module 4, so this module will focus on stress management, exercise, physiology, sleep and the mind/thinking habits that all are correlated with each other. As Dr. Andrew Weil says, you need to attend to all lifestyle factors that relate to healthy aging – how you eat, your physical activity, how you handle stress, sleep and relationships. You need to focus on all those areas in order to have proper balance.

STRESS is the worst toxin in the entire body that affects your thoughts, feelings and behavior, and makes your energy off-balance. Stress, hard work, and lots of thinking create tension in the body, which can lead to chronic aches, stiffness, and constipation. If left unchecked, stress can contribute to major health problems, such as high blood pressure, heart disease, obesity and diabetes.

How to cope with stress

- **Have downtime! Treat yourself!** • Go for a walk, practice yoga, listen to music, meditate, get a massage. This helps to clear your head. *Tip: Use the meditation and 1½-minute breathing exercises introduced in Module 2.*
- **Get enough sleep.** • When stressed, your body needs additional sleep and rest. *Tip: Try to take naps on weekends to catch up on sleep.*
- **Move your body daily** • to help you feel good and maintain your health. This doesn't mean hard-core exercise. Studies show that just 30 minutes of physical activity every other day is all that's required to reap big benefits.
- **Keep your diet balanced** • Proper nutrition reduces stress.
- **Do more enjoyable things** • Just enjoying yourself will help you reduce the levels of stress hormones cortisol and epinephrine. For example, volunteering gives you a break from everyday stress and makes you "feel good."

We all have some level of stress, so learning to cope with it is the first step. However, we do need to understand ways to reduce it because, over time, it can cause major health problems. Learn what triggers your anxiety and do something about it.

PRACTICAL TOOL 5-1: Stress Reduction	
My stress triggers are: (describe the trigger)	What could I do differently to overcome that trigger?
Commute:	
Work:	
Family:	
Children:	
Finances:	
Health:	
School:	
Relationship:	
Other:	

We often are too busy to think about what actually makes us stressed out, but this is the source of all evil in our lives. You can diet, exercise, breathe, treat yourself all you want, but if you don't address stress triggers, nothing will change in your life. Once you solve the source of a problem, your life will change for the better. Hopefully, this exercise has made you aware of what is causing the stress, so you can start taking actions to make your life more enjoyable. Life is too short; let's make every day count.

PHYSICAL ACTIVITY is incredibly important for keeping your energy balanced which, in turn, leads to balanced overall health and well-being. When you go for a walk or work out, there are many benefits:

- You burn calories.
- You build muscle mass, which increases your metabolism. *Tip: Each pound of lean muscle burns an additional 25-50 calories every day for the rest of your life.*
- Hormones are balanced in your body.
- Your immune system improves.
- You detoxify your body through perspiring.
- Endorphins get released, making you feel excited, energized and happy.
- You will have increased energy.
- You even slow the aging process as you improve skin and muscle tone.
- You will sleep better. *Tip: Studies have shown that moderate to vigorous 20- to 30-minute workouts three to four times a week help you sleep better.* The quality of your sleep improve, too.
- As you get toned, you will look better and have more self-confidence. *Tip: New opportunities open up; it all starts from within.*
- Exercise makes your brain function at its best. You will experience improved memory, reaction time and concentration.

So if you haven't been walking or exercising before, this list should help change your mind. There are too many benefits to leave on the table. So let's get moving and have some fun!

When it comes to physical activity, everybody chooses what works for them best. There are strength training, cardio (walking, jogging, cycling, spinning, tennis etc.), flexibility and balance (Pilates, yoga), martial arts, wrestling, skiing, rowing, paddle boarding, surfing, kayaking, golfing etc. We all have our own preferences that fit our body type and energy levels. Some of us like competitive team sports, others prefer to exercise solo. There is no right or wrong; whatever feels right, is the right way. The most important thing is to move your body and do things you enjoy. This is the only way to make it part of your life – not just because it is good for you, but because you like it. Remember, like attracts like, so the more enjoyable things you do, the more enjoyable things you receive.

Regardless of what exercise you like, to reach your full potential physically, you need to use a **mindfulness technique** used by many professional athletes, including Olympic teams. The key is to step back, relax, become aware of the moment and focus on the exercise you are doing, i.e. visualize the ball going where it needs to go and it is more likely to go there. This mindfulness technique is a time-tested way to winning!

By focusing and concentrating on what you are doing, you are able to flex your muscles to their full potential – not too much and not too little. The body moves naturally and to the best of its ability. When you look back, you probably notice how most sports injuries happened when you have been distracted and something caught you off-guard. I have hurt my lower back doing yoga only when I have been distracted by thinking about something and not paying attention to the alignment, because yoga is all about perfect alignment, perfect balance. When your mind is off-balance, your body also will be off-balance. Working out mindfully will maximize your workout and keep you fit and safe.

Once you have your mind ready, it is time to set some goals and develop a fitness routine that delivers those goals. Don't forget to capture current and real-istic target weight goals as well as body measurements (waist, thighs, hips, chest), because muscle weighs more than fat. *Tip: It is a good idea to add workouts to your calendar so they don't end up getting moved around or canceled.*

PRACTICAL TOOL 5-2: My Fitness Program

Key Steps:

1. What are your fitness goals, i.e. weight loss, health, energy, strength, flexibility, balance, etc.?

2. How much time can you allocate for exercise per week and when, i.e. weekend warrior, or early mornings or evenings, etc.?

3. Self-Assessment: How fit are you? Choose a plan that fits your level.

4. Do you have any health issues, i.e. high blood pressure? Listen to your body. You can put together a menu of activities to keep yourself in balance, i.e. if you are stressed out, choose a more calming, relaxing exercise like yoga or swimming.

5. What activities do you enjoy? Develop a plan that you love. Think about what you loved to do as a kid. What will get you moving?

6. Monitor your progress and adjust, if needed.

Once you have set your goals, the program you choose could vary considerably. For example, you probably have heard that, if you want to lose weight, it is 80% dependent on what you eat and 20% on exercise. Regardless of the goal, everybody knows that exercise is good for you, but time is always the key barrier. There just aren't enough hours in a day to do everything. When I was in the corporate world, all that mattered to me was how I could achieve the most in the least amount of time. I will share here what worked for me and has proven to work for most people.

Based on my experience, the most optimum weight loss exercise routine is a combination of cardio (jogging, biking, tennis, etc.) and strength training (lifting weights) for achieving ideal body weight. Cardio exercise will help you burn many calories short-term, while strength training builds your muscle for long-term calorie burning by increasing your metabolism. It is important to note that, beginning at age 25, we lose 5 pounds of muscle mass every 10 years. So, naturally, a combination of both – cardio (short-) and strength (long-term) – will maximize your calorie-burning power and your fitness level. However, this combination exercise schedule tends to consume quite a lot of time that busy professionals don't have, i.e. alternating cardio three times a week with strength three times a week (30-minute+ sessions each).

When time is a limiting factor, the most effective and efficient workout seems to be a **High Intensity Interval Training (HIIT)**. Besides being a quick method to getting in a great workout, intervals are extremely effective for transforming your physique. HIIT consists of short, intense bursts of exercise, followed by low-intensity exercise or complete rest in-between. Intense circuits not only help you build lean muscle mass, but also help develop the cardio-vascular system. By pushing your heart rate high during periods of work, you'll increase your cardio ability and strengthen your heart. A perfect combination of strength and cardio is definitely a win, win! To jump-start your routine, just Google "high intensity interval workouts" or "HIIT workouts" and pick one or two to incorporate into your weekly routine. Include at least a day of rest in-between workouts, as these intervals are intense. The entire HIIT session may last between 4 (four) and 30 minutes, meaning that it is considered to be an excellent way to maximize a workout that is limited by time[2]. Depending on your objectives, combine exercises, tools and time intervals to obtain the optimal result.

In case HIIT is not for you, don't get discouraged. My dad is in his 60's and, honestly, I don't see him doing jumping jacks. He does strength training three times a week at the gym, coupled with occasional short walks when he feels like it, and he has lost 30 pounds in few months and is successfully maintaining his weight. The key is to follow the right eating habits and, when exercising, to exhaust each muscle group to the point that you cannot make any more repetitions. Whatever you choose to do, it is important that it becomes part of your weekly schedule. That's the only way you see results. While you are exercising, do not forget to hydrate yourself. Based on studies, 85% of headaches happen because of dehydration.

Ideally, we want to make "moving" a part of our lifestyle. As Dr. John J. Ratey, associate clinical professor of psychiatry at Harvard Medical School, says: "From your genes to your emotions, your body and brain are dying to embrace the physical life. You are built to move. When you do, you'll be on fire! "Whether that's cycling to work, walking the dog, stepping up your walking pace, taking the stairs instead of the elevator, parking your car at the rear end of the parking lot or doing push-ups during the breaks for ads on TV, it is all about moving your body, and that's what our bodies are meant to be doing. This becomes especially important when you are sitting in front of the computer all day long.

Finally, most of us need about 7 to 8 hours of sleep a night for optimal rest, fat loss and muscle growth. When I was part of the corporate world, I remember how it wasn't always easy to get a good night's sleep; I had so many ideas and thoughts running around in my head, falling asleep often was one of the hardest things to do. Our hyperactive minds are strongly linked with sleeplessness. Sleep is a hormone-dependent process and, with all the variables in our lives that can affect proper hormone balance (foods, exercise, stress, etc.), it makes sense that many people struggle with sleep. There is a strong relationship between chronic illnesses and sleep.

Simple tricks to improve your sleep

- Wake up and go to bed at the same time, even on weekends, to keep your hormone cycle regular.
- Eat a high-protein snack a few hours before going to bed (before 7 p.m.).
- Avoid caffeine after 2 p.m.
- Drink chamomile tea. Chamomile works as a mild tranquilizer and a sleep inducer.
- Avoid alcohol at night because, initially, it serves as a stimulant and then affects the nervous system and makes you feel depressed. It can affect the REM cycle, meaning you could be waking up in the middle of the night.
- The ideal room temperature for sleeping is 65°-68° Fahrenheit. Cooling the room will decrease your core body temperature and induce sleepiness.
- When you make your muscles more relaxed, you will feel more relaxed. Take a soothing sea-salt bath or a hot shower about an hour before going to bed with a great book or some relaxing music playing in the background.
- Use blackout curtains when possible and turn off all night lights that might spoil the darkness. Melatonin cannot keep us asleep whenever there is light.
- Get at least 30 minutes of sunlight each day. The exposure to the sun during the day boosts serotonin levels, which will help improve melatonin levels at night.
- Try not to exercise hard two hours before going to bed. Stretching is beneficial; it will help you relax your muscles without raising your heart rate before sleep.
- Meditate or do the 1½-minute breathing exercise introduced in Module 2. It's all about calming our minds. *Note: My dad has been using the 1½-minute breathing exercise (4-7-8) before bedtime and it really works like magic. He sleeps like a baby!*

To summarize: We need it all – good mind, good nutrition, good physical activity and good sleep in order to have good energy balance that leads to good health and good life. It is important to focus on beating stress and body imbalances that affect the quality of our sleep and health. When we lead busy lives, it takes a major commitment to health and well-being, but when you know your body changes shape and when attitudes transform as you embrace the holistic, incredibly effective body and mind lifestyle, it'll all be worth it in the end.

As your mind becomes strong and fit, your body will become strong and fit, leading to perfect alignment and energy balance.

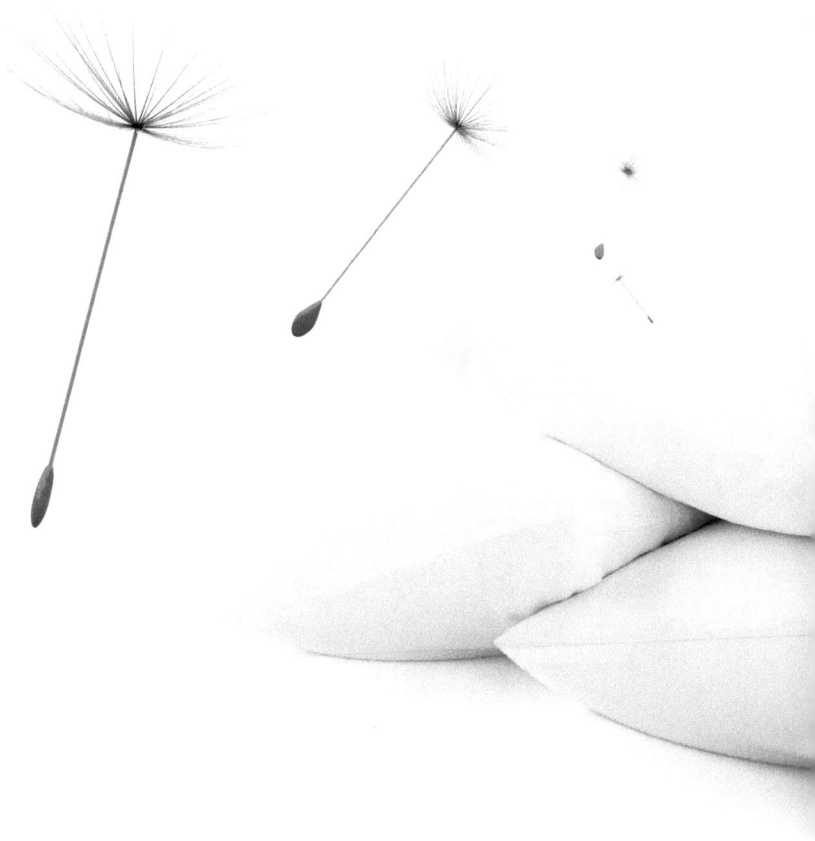

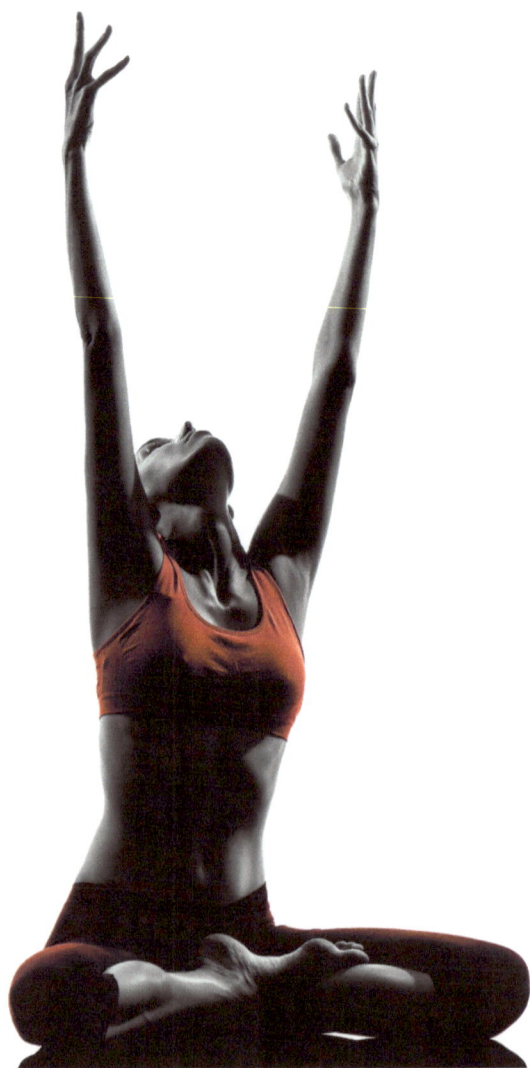

module

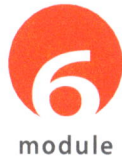

GOOD BODY: LOOK GOOD

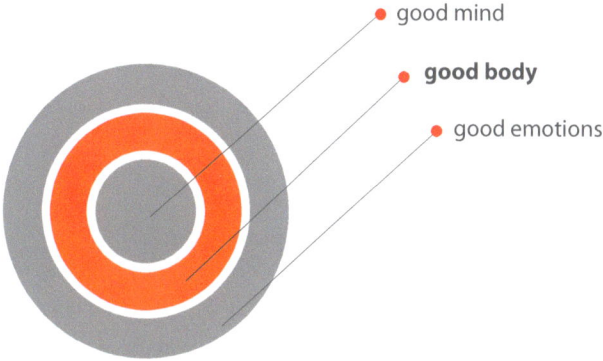

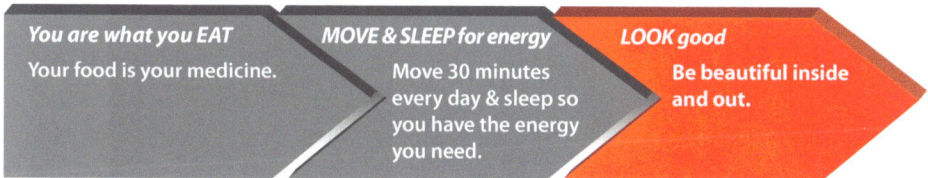

good mind

good body

good emotions

You are what you EAT
Your food is your medicine.

MOVE & SLEEP for energy
Move 30 minutes every day & sleep so you have the energy you need.

LOOK good
Be beautiful inside and out.

Be beautiful inside and out.

We live in the physical world. Like attracts like. So be the person you want to meet or like the people who you'd want to surround you. Respect yourself, take care of yourself and look the part. Figure out who you are and what makes you unique; what your style should be so your unique personality can come through and shine.

This concept actually is not that different from building global billion-dollar brands. It is all about figuring out who we are and for what we stand. What makes us unique and different from anybody else. What our best parts are and how we can make them stand out. Who is our target market, and why they should buy our brand rather than our competitor's. This is exactly what we need to do with our personal identity.

We need to figure out our own PERSONAL IDENTITY. Who we are and how we want to show ourselves to the world. But let's not get confused by image, because that is how people actually perceive us and the image we portray. Ideally, we want both the IDENTITY and IMAGE aligned, otherwise there is a disconnect between who we think we are and how others perceive us, which will make "selling" ourselves more difficult. There are times when we actually need to re-brand ourselves. This often happens when we are going through a significant change in our lives. We finally discover that who we have been is no longer who we want to be and it is time to shed that old skin so the new bright skin can shine through.

One of my clients had this experience. After working with her for three months, her thinking evolved and her perspectives changed. When your perspectives change, your reality changes. So she suddenly realized that her Miami Beach style is not who she is anymore. She has grown up, she is empowered to do amazing things and that confidence, that feeling comfortable in her own skin needs to come through. She completely changed her wardrobe to urban chic and she stepped into the world as a new shining star.

Like good marketers do, let's now create our PERSONAL IDENTITY or, as it is called in the brand world, the Unique Selling Proposition (USP). This sentence is not just a sentence, but your DNA, your reason for being. Think about for what you stand and what sets you apart. Write it down into a sentence.

PRACTICAL TOOL 6-1: My Personal Identity

My name is _____. I love _____.
I didn't like _____. So I created _____ that _____.

This statement sums up the WHAT you do, the WHY you do it and the WHY someone else should care about it. Give it a try and see what comes up!

Another important part of BRANDING is the look and feel. In our case, the style. STYLE is a form of self-expression. You could be whoever you choose to be. The most important thing is to BE YOU and stay true to yourself without trying to fit into the same mold as everybody else. You know you have the right Personal Identity/the right Style when you feel comfortable and confident – that sensation of being "unstoppable," "this is so me." There are many ways to describe different styles, beginning with chic, couture, elegant, bold, sporty, glam, sophisticated, nautical, earthy, polished, urban, classic, statement, vintage, etc., and ending with masculine, feminine. They all are amazing styles in their own right. The key is to find the right style for you. It is quite normal that we go through an evolution of fashion throughout our lives as the trends change, but most of those changes are linked to us changing, becoming more in tune with who we are. Below is a simple exercise to figure out how you would describe your style and then looking to see if your outfits actually match that style. If not, it may be time for a closet makeover, so you can not only "be you," but "look you."

PRACTICAL TOOL 6-2: My Style Guide

Who is my fashion icon, i.e. Jackie Kennedy Onassis, Sarah Jessica Parker, Kate Middleton, Tiger Woods, Victoria and David Beckham, etc.?

Where do I usually shop, i.e. Zara, Banana Republic, Elie Tahari, Brooks Brothers, etc.?

What's my favorite outfit, i.e. makes me feel most comfortable?

What are my favorite accessories, i.e. belts, scarves, jewelry or less is more?

What colors do I like to wear? Earthy neutral tones or vivid ones?

How would I describe my style? Choose from: sporty, casual, urban, chic, elegant, classic, modern, glam, couture, bold, sophisticated, nautical, earthy, polished, statement, vintage

Do the clothes in the closet match the style I WANT to have as compared to WHAT I have?

Your style, your self-expression is the first impression the world gets of you, so be your best. They often say that, when you go to interviews, the interviewer makes his or her hiring decision within the first few minutes, so it is all about that first impression. When it comes to first impressions, obviously it is so much more than just the outfit you are wearing. It is how you wear it, your body language, a strong handshake, being polite and well-mannered, making eye contact, being articulate, etc.

Now that we know our IDENTITY and STYLE, let us turn to beauty. We all know true beauty starts from within. When we feel beautiful, we are beautiful. When we are happy and joyful, kind and loving, the room fills with grace and we are truly beautiful inside and outside. When we feel depressed, unhappy, sleep-deprived or stressed out, it will be hard to see beauty around us. It all comes back to our mind. Our mind controls everything.

Beauty does literally start from within. You could constantly be hunting for the latest innovation, anti-aging skincare and hair-care products to get those beauty results you have been desiring. But the truth is, those products treat the symptoms, not the cause. Don't get me wrong, cleaning, exfoliating, clarifying, moisturizing your skin, plus using sunscreen, are important daily beauty routines, but we are only touching the surface. The real beauty starts from the foods we eat. With the proper nourishment and care, our body stays youthful and vibrant.

We are what we eat. Even the most expensive skin cream isn't going to do anything for you unless your are supplying your body with the nutrition it needs to look beautiful. Collagen controls our skin elasticity, so we need to keep those levels high. When food gets processed to create energy, free radicals are produced that are highly-charged oxygen molecules and are harmful to the skin. They are usually neutralized by antioxidants like vitamins C, E, etc. However, when the body is overwhelmed by free radicals, and supply of antioxidants is limited, wrinkling of the skin may occur. The most common causes of free radicals are excess sun, smoking, stress and obesity. The more free radicals you have, the more likely it is that you will look older than you are. When you eat junk and processed foods, your skin is going to look dull, dry and aged. From the moment you first start eating nutritious food, your skin will start showing signs of renewal. So it is never too early to start.

Here are those beauty super foods

• **Hot water with lemon** • a long-time beauty staple to hydrate and detoxify your body. Have a glass of hot water with lemon first thing when you wake up and you will see and feel the difference.

• **Green tea** • a magical tea that is filled not only with antioxidants that help neutralize free radicals to help your skin remain youthful and radiant, but also flushes out toxins, eases bloating and increases your metabolism. Ideally, replace your coffee with green tea, but if that's not possible, then even just one cup of green tea a day will work wonders.

• **Almonds** • contain important antioxidants, nutrients like Omega 3 fatty acids, protein, vitamin E, magnesium and calcium that are essential for healthy skin and hair. The more antioxidants you have in your diet, the more likely you will be able to preserve your youthful appearance. Have at least 5 almonds a day!

• **Coconut oil** • a multi-functional beauty staple used for cooking, hair, skin, sunscreen, a natural appetite suppressant. It can be applied to the face as a mois-turizer or used as a sunscreen.

• **Spinach** • rich in folic acid that helps convert our food into usable energy. This gives you that natural glow and offers a variety of restorative and youth-enhancing benefits.

• **Celery** • packed with nutrients like vitamins A and C, and alkaline minerals like magnesium and reduce stress levels. High in antioxidants that help fight free radicals that have accumulated in your body.

• **Papaya** • often used in beauty products because of its strong antioxidant power in fighting free radicals. High in folic acid, and contains enzyme that helps with digestion.

• **Tomatoes** • our favorite kitchen staple offers numerous health and beauty benefits. Tomatoes are one of the most powerful super foods in getting rid of signs of sun damage. Packed with vitamins like A, K and B; minerals like iron, magnesium and phosphorus.

• **Salmon** • filled with nutrients aiding in better brain function, thicker, fuller hair and even clearer skin because it includes Omega 3 fatty acids, DHA and EPA (both highly unsaturated fats). Try to have salmon a couple of times a week.

• **Red kidney beans** • full of iron, protein, magnesium, and many other anti-oxidants that can help your body prevent diseases, neutralize free radicals and help enhance the look and feel of your skin. Contains zinc, a mineral that can help repair skin and hair damage, and a nutrient called biotin that is essential for growing healthy and strong nails.

• **Oysters, lobster** • good sources of zinc, which aids in skin cell renewal and repair. Zinc also keeps your nails, hair and eyes healthy.

• **Blueberries** • particularly rich in flavones which have anti-inflammatory and antioxidant properties, protecting you from premature aging, and your skin from sun damage.

• **Bell peppers** • their high vitamin C content kicks up collagen production for healthy hair and skin.

• **Sweet potatoes** • packed with beta-carotene, an antioxidant that fights aging.

Super foods packed with antioxidants can raise your beauty to the next level; they also contribute to glowing skin, weight loss, better sleep, better ability to deal with stress and make you more energetic and balanced. Your biological age can drop by 10 years. We really are what we eat.

In order to maximize our anti-aging power, we need to think beyond food. We want to take care of our body through nutrition, sleep, rest and exercise that will leave the skin, mind and energy restored. There is no magic bullet to anti-aging. Anti-aging is a process toward which you work your entire life. It's a lifestyle change for which you must be ready.

A good example is my friend in New York City. She is in her 30's and living an amazing life. She is always on the go, working hard, often socializing – which involves drinking. One day, she called, telling me how she is making a deliberate effort to live a healthier life. She told me that she hasn't had any alcohol for the past nine days, is making healthy home-cooked meals rather than eating out all the time, and is exercising regularly. As a result, her skin has cleared up and she is sleeping better. She even said how her mind is clearer and, for some reason, she feels happier. I was very pleased to hear all about her quick wins and explained how it only gets better.

There is a point in everybody's life when it is time to choose what kind of life you would like to live and how you would like to look and feel. I often worry about people who burn the candle at both ends.

The key aging factors are stress, free radical levels, muscle elasticity and hormone levels. Once we keep those factors under control and balanced, we will maximize our beauty and youthfulness.

To summarize: To LOOK GOOD, we need to take care of our body and mind. We have reviewed how to define our own Personal Identity – who we are and what makes us unique. We understand our Personal Style and what makes us feel good – comfortable and confident. Beauty starts from within. When we feel beautiful, we are beautiful. With the right nutrition and healthy lifestyle habits, you will feel your best. You will feel more youthful, energetic and happy, coupled with self-confidence and self-esteem, knowing that you are just as beautiful on the inside as you are on the outside.

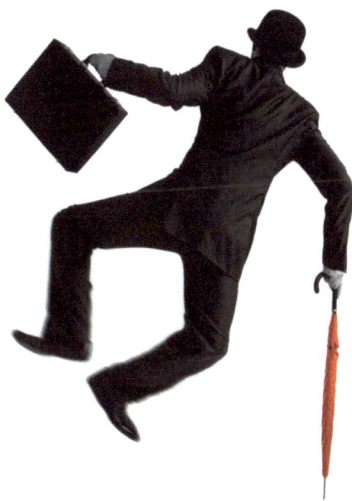

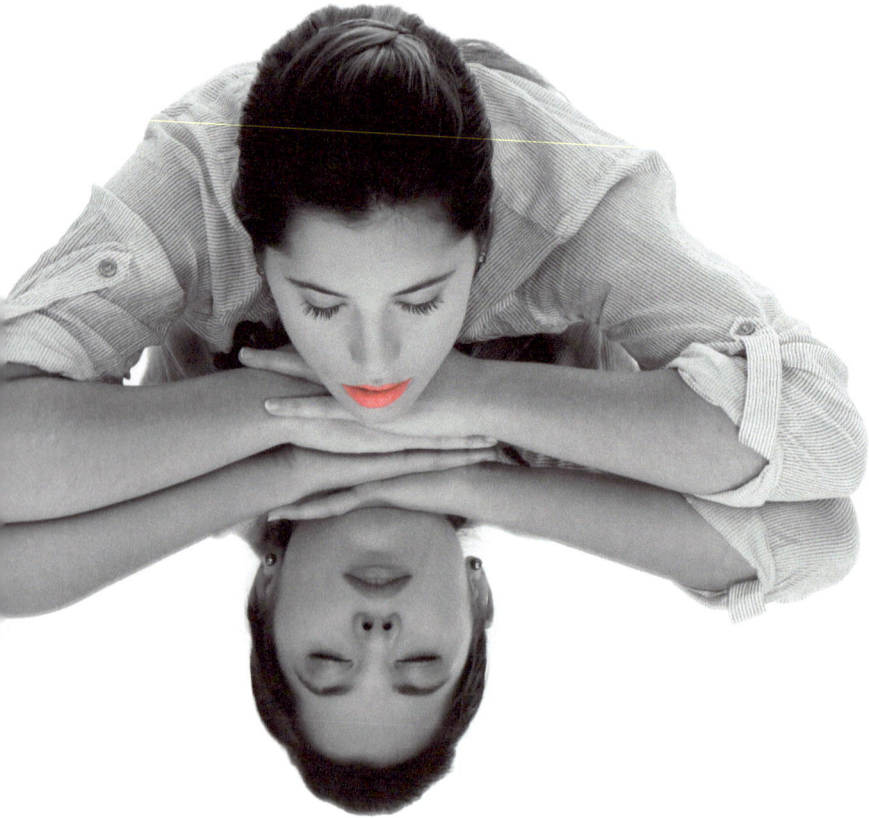

7

module

GOOD EMOTIONS: BE THE BEST YOU

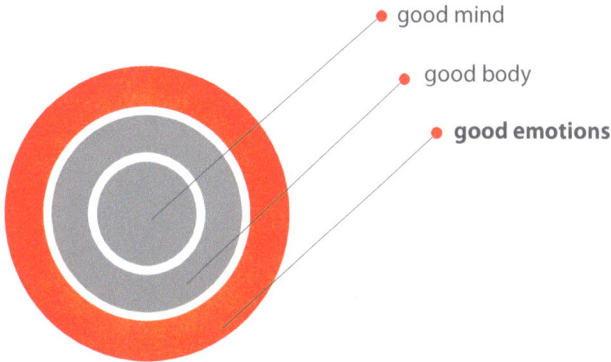

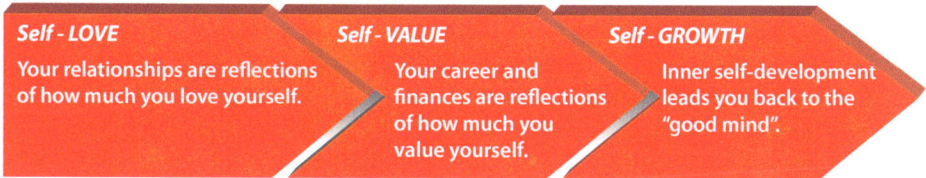

● good mind

● good body

● **good emotions**

Self - LOVE	*Self - VALUE*	*Self - GROWTH*
Your relationships are reflections of how much you love yourself.	Your career and finances are reflections of how much you value yourself.	Inner self-development leads you back to the "good mind".

You are the mirror of your life.

Our emotional state and well-being is the most important part of our lives. It's how we actually FEEL; it's the love, joy, sadness and all other emotions. Our emotions are a direct result of how we treat our mind and body. That's why, in this module, we have no practical tools, since all the work already has been done and it's time to reap the rewards. When we treat our body well – properly nourished, well-rested, fit and filled with energy – our emotions will be positive. We feel happy and joyful. When we treat our body like it's the least important thing on our agenda – malnourished, sleep-deprived and stressed out – our emotions will be negative. That's the reason why we need to take care of our mind and body. Mind, body and emotions are integrally linked; one affects the other. When you have/display an angry emotion, you most likely will feel pain in your physical body as well. When your thoughts are negative, your energy vibration goes down, attracting more unhappy emotions. When you think of uplifting things, your energy vibration goes up, attracting more positive feelings and emotions.

The truth is, it is quite challenging always to be positive, but at least we should do our best to see a glimpse of light even when everything looks gloomy. I remember the story about a man who had no reason to be positive about anything, but thought, as he often retells it now, "Okay, let me try this gratitude and positive thinking stuff to see if it really works." It did! There are many success stories where gratitude has led to abundance, emotionally as well as physically.

You are the mirror of your life. How you treat yourself, others will treat you. Your relationships reflect how much you love yourself. Every relationship self-help book I have ever read stresses the same thing: When you begin VALUING YOURSELF, loving the way you look, doing things that are good for you and make you happy, appreciating your precious time and respecting your existence, the right partner somehow magically shows up. Your energy attracts a partner who vibrates on the same wavelength. Your beliefs define how much you love, honor and respect yourself. Your relationships will reflect that state of mind. If you feel that "I am not good enough," then you are looking for someone to make you feel complete. When things change, the relationship could fall apart. A true bond can be built only on a strong foundation, when two people are complete in their own right. We want to be with people who lift us up, not push us down. Life is too short to waste it on anything but the utmost good.

The same is true with your career and finances. Both are a reflection of how much you value yourself – your SELF-WORTH. If you are not happy with yourself, you don't feel confident, and that lack of confidence holds you back from success and financial gain.

To illustrate how this works, I'll share the story of one of my clients. When we started working together, my client was in a very unhappy place and felt as though there was something blocking her getting what she really wanted. Being the outsider looking in, I saw that all of her energy was spent on working

24/7 and she did nothing to take care of herself – her health, her well-being – other than yo-yo dieting and taking some pills. We started working on her life's goals, passions, talents, nutrition, exercise, sleep, prioritizing her workload and other lifestyle habits and, most importantly, bringing more joy into her life; that included doing things she loves, i.e. walks in the park, attending art exhibitions, joining fitness club, meditating, etc. As we began introducing all the new, enjoyable, "good for her" things into her life, her stress level dropped and the weight started to fall off naturally. Once her weight changed (being the major block), she had a complete wardrobe makeover and picked a new, more appropriate style to match her new empowering self-assurance. Because of her confidence and respect for her body, mind and spirit, she started attracting love and romance, something that had been missing from her life for years. She now has a boyfriend and is in a happy relationship. Because she looks so good inside and out, she has been given an opportunity to fulfill one of her biggest dreams. Her words, "Overall health, well-being and image give me the confidence I need to rise in my career and step in front of millions of people. Without that, I wouldn't even be thinking about it." Once she started to value herself and take care of herself, her self-worth increased and all those new money-making opportunities now are available to her. And as she truly loves the way she looks and feels presently, she is attracting romantic relationships. Like energy attracts like energy. All it takes is to remove the blocks from life's path and life begins to follow the course you create through your goals and manifestation.

Our purpose in life is to live and grow intellectually and spiritually. Constant learning, SELF-GROWTH, will keep our brain fit and strong. Our brain is constantly making connections. As new information comes into our brain, we start making new connections and creating new thoughts and ideas and taking new actions. And new, amazing things start to happen. It's all about taking little steps, i.e. explore a new neighborhood, shop in a new grocery store, try a new cuisine or recipe, etc. When we keep knowing and doing the same old thing, nothing will change in our lives.

We are all born with a magical life. It is our birth right. We are born with our gifts, talents and passions for a reason: so we all could contribute something amazing to this world. Otherwise we all would be exactly the same. Frequently those gifts and talents come so naturally to us that we take them for granted, but others definitely take notice. Because we don't have to work hard for those talents, we undervalue them and don't use them in any meaningful way. As a result, we end up doing something we are not meant to be doing, something at which we need to work hard, often taking a toll on our health, and life in general, and paying a heavy price for it in the end. Whether it is a failed marriage or heart failure. However, when we recognize and accept our gifts and talents, we can see that the key to our success and happiness is inside ourselves – not in the ones we think we are suppose to be.

We all also begin as pure love, and then the "stories" start happening, i.e. we experience hurt, pain, fear, anger, etc., and that conditions us to feel and think a certain way, and it becomes our belief. Someone may have betrayed you and, because of that circumstance, you are likely to experience trust issues. Your parents may have divorced when you were a child and, because of that experience, you may now be overprotective of your heart so nobody can hurt you, and the list continues. These stories/blocks/beliefs define our actions and who we are. It becomes a list of rules, interests, titles, labels (I am a father, a vice president, a golfer, etc.); but those are just expressions and not really who we are. Many of us are building houses on shaky foundations because we do not know who we are.

Do you know anybody whose life seems magical? How they always manage to be calm and effortlessly manage their busy lives? Wonderful things happen to them and their lives are filled with love, joy and prosperity. And you wonder if they were born under a lucky star. Truth is, we all are born under a lucky star, but how we choose to see and live our lives defines success or failure, happiness or unhappiness. That choice is often based on our "stories." Our perspectives define our reality.

We all are looking for a purpose. Our purpose is to live life. Everything we do should have a purpose. Instead of making a decision, we often analyze and over-think things. Listen to your inner guidance, your gut feeling, and you won't go wrong. Get out of your head and get into your heart. Fear is often our biggest enemy, stopping us from pursuing our dreams. It is inherently connected to our "stories," and that's one of the main reasons why we end up staying where we are. People spend a lot more time avoiding what they don't want to have rather than going after what they want. What are you afraid of? What is taking up a lot of that space of your mind and time? Get out of that comfort zone, where the underlying feeling is fear and not knowing what will happen. Not knowing is the most exciting part of living! A leap of faith is all it takes to move on.

We want to drop those "stories" by just changing the words we use, because "what I say is who I become." To bring this to life, if you are constantly late to meetings, then probably you're late for many things in life. It shows low self-esteem. The point is, stay true to your words, because you are what you say, what you do.

To summarize: The source of all being is SELF-CARE. Be in love with yourself! Be the best expression of health and vitality. Stop worrying about other people; be present and self-honoring, and that's when inner guidance can come in. Follow your inner guidance. Take a step and take another step – show up! Being THE BEST VERSION OF YOU is a process, a step-by-step journey – not a destination nor an event.

> There are two basic motivating forces:
> fear and love. When we are afraid,
> we pull back from life.
> When we are in love, we open to all
> that life has to offer with passion,
> excitement, and acceptance.
> We need to learn to love ourselves first,
> in all our glory and our imperfections.
> If we cannot love ourselves,
> we cannot fully open to our ability
> to love others or our potential to create.
> Evolution and all hopes
> for a better world rest in
> the fearlessness and open-hearted vision of
> people who embrace life.
>
> – John Lennon

conclusion

Our life's purpose is to find ourselves and to realize our full potential.

I believe there are three basic aspects to life – body, mind and emotions. The fourth is the spirit that, indirectly, we have addressed in this guide. I wanted to create something which nurtures all three aspects to achieve a deeper, more sophisticated level of well-being. There aren't too many options out there addressing emotions and mind in tandem with body and, to some extent, spirit. This guide has pulled it all together so you can have a one-stop shop to "good health. good life."

Consider this guide to be an investment, and a very worthy one, in yourself. If you can learn how to make yourself a priority and embrace it through healthy living and truly good habits, then you have uncovered what it takes. We simply need to get into the rhythm of life, which is slow and purposeful rather than rushed and hectic. Ultimately, the point is to figure out our own personal program, a winning formula that can be integrated into our life at home, at work and in the midst of a daily routine. There are many benefits to this holistic approach to wellness: it offers guidance and practical tools needed to age happily and healthily. Exercise, nutrition, stress management and other lifestyle habits all play a role in healthy living and directly impacting your emotional well-being and your relationships.

It can be quite difficult to change a lifelong habit or deal with stress and still maintain a healthy daily routine, but extra help is at hand. Destination spas, retreats and many coaching practices are now attending to clients' physical and emotional issues, and offering fitness guidance as well as aesthetic treatments. You are never alone!

To sum up, there are some key principles of "good health. good life." that will help you live a beautiful life:

• **"If you love something, set it free!"** • Often, we try to control a person or a circumstance and wonder why they keep pulling away. If you let go and set it free, everything falls in the right place naturally.

• **"What you resist, persists."** • In other words, if you focus on something, it becomes real. So if you keep thinking about "lack of money," that's what most likely you'll experience. Thinking about gratitude and how much you already have now almost certainly will increase your abundance.

• **"Release attachment to result."** • As Buddha says, "A problem cannot cause suffering. It is our thinking and attachment to it that causes suffering." Sometimes we want something that may not be the best thing for us. Remember to have faith. Believe everything happens for a reason and that there is a higher purpose that is so much better than we can imagine and, suddenly, life gets a lot easier.

• **There are two sides, "success and failure," to everything in life.** • How you choose to see the world determines your success or failure. So be grateful and positive!

• **"Fear is excitement on 'pause'. "** • Before every great deed, fear is always present.

• **Take a leap of faith!** • It is important to have faith and believe that everything works out as it should. We do not need to control our lives; just let go and enjoy the ride.

• **Make a different choice to get a different result.** • Take action toward the new choice. The outside world is a reflection of the choices we have made inside.

• **It all comes together when you figure out who you are.** • You are the only relationship about which you have to worry. That relationship is being reflected in your life – loving you, knowing you within. In all the experiences of life, you are the common denominator.

• **Life is not easy.** • As Dr. Bernie Siegel, a retired general/pediatric surgeon and published author, says, "We have to create perfection through love. It is a weapon. When someone is driving you crazy, tell them, 'I love you.' They don't know what to say. Saves you a lot of therapy!"

There is one suggestion I would like to offer all the parents out there; it's one that will make your children's lives extraordinary and this world a better place. Love your children like there is no tomorrow! All the values and beliefs, those "stories" that define us, are formed during childhood, so be there for your children to provide them with the best possible life and guidance. Do protect them; however, encourage their creativity, joy, freedom and wisdom. Guide them wisely so they discover who they are and what they love in life. Don't force someone else's box on them. Love them and set them free!

We have come to the end of this guide, but to the start of a new beginning: "good health. good life." Do your best to make your life extraordinary, truly spectacular! You are exactly where you are meant to be. Don't worry so much; most of the things are out of your control. You are the only relationship about which you have to think. Forgive, "rewrite" the past, and focus on all the good in your life. When you live your life from the heart, you never can go wrong. Choose to be in the place of peace, joy and prosperity, surrounded by people who lift you up and fill your heart. Use those gifts and share that love that you have received. Open your heart to the people who treat you well and wish all the best for those who don't. Be grateful for what you have and enjoy the now – the only time that has been granted to you. Love your life and all the beauty that surrounds you. Life is a privilege, so make it beautiful, make it count.

May you always be blessed with good health and good life.
Love & Light!

They say, "When you learn to dance, you can finally hear the music!" I say, "When you learn to live, you can finally see the beauty!"

– Helen Marie Loorents

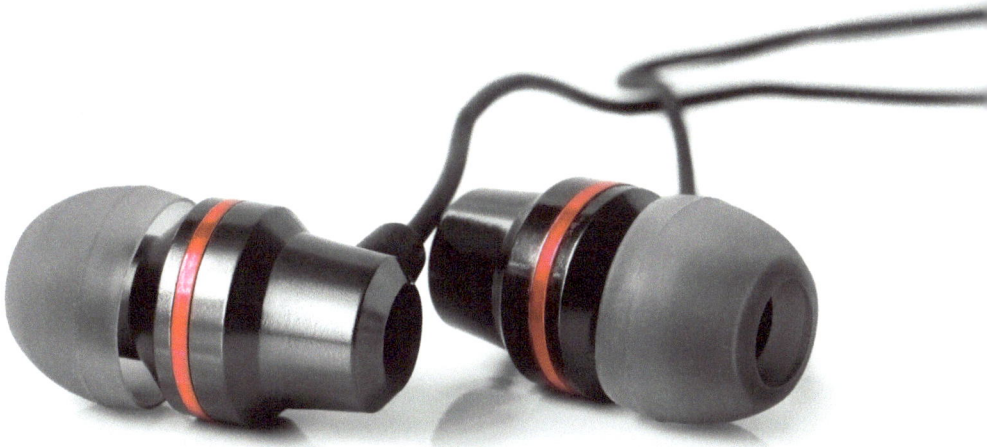

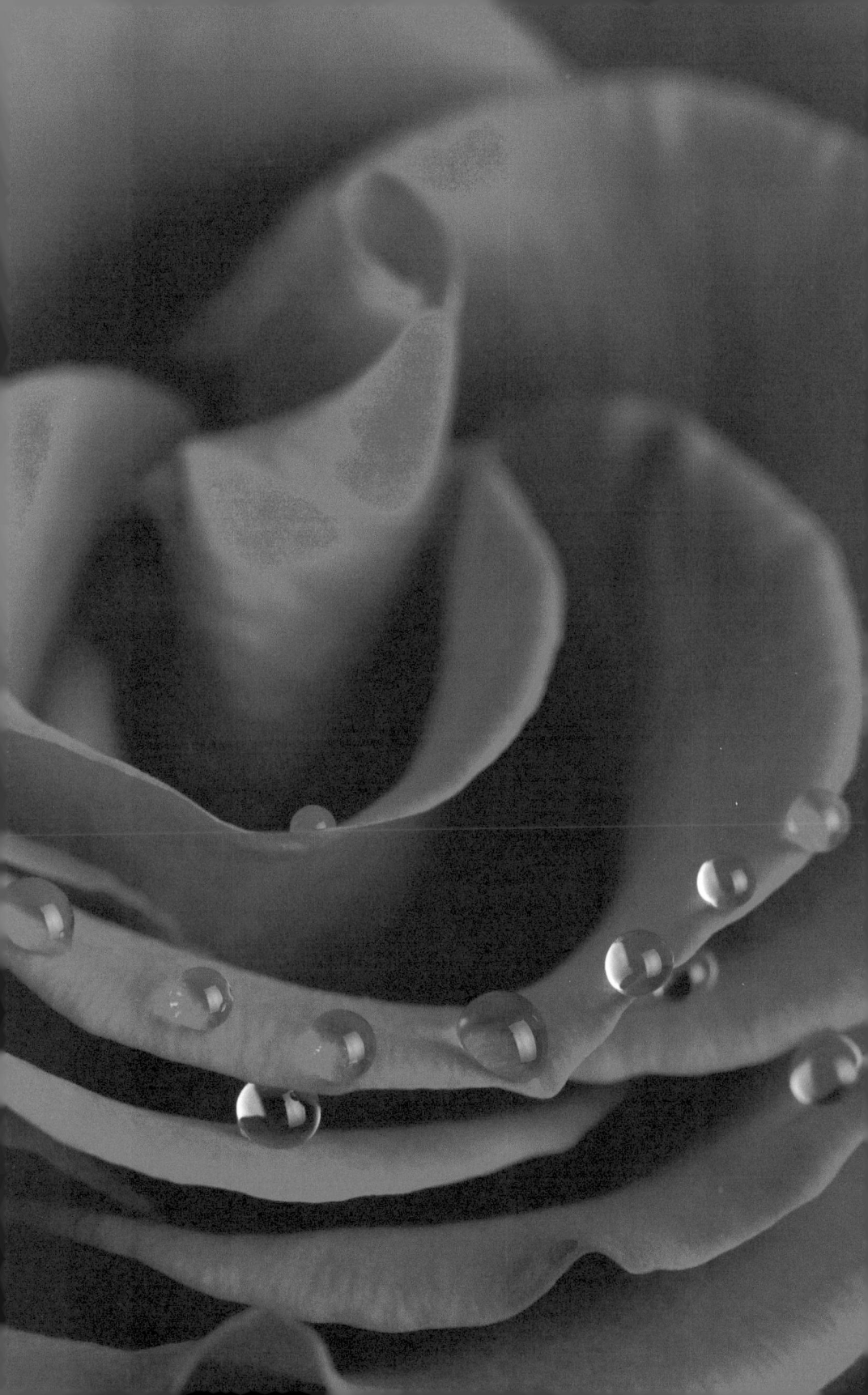

bibliography

[1] Lally, Phillippa, Cornelia H.M. Van Jaarsveld, Henry W.W. Potts, and Jane Wardle. "How Are Habits Formed: Modeling Habit Formation in the Real World." European Journal of Social Psychology Volume 40, Issue 6, Pages 998-1009, October 2010, 16 July 2009. Web. 14 August 2014.

[2] Van Dusen, Allison (Oct. 20, 2008). "Ten ways to get more from your workout". Forbes. Retrieved Dec. 14, 2008.

Organizations

Institute for the Integrative Nutrition
3 E 28th St, New York, NY 10016
(877) 730-5444
www.integrativenutrition.com

Dr. Jacqueline Sidman, PhD, president
The Sidman Institute, Irvine, CA
(949) 553-0621
www.sidmansolution.com

Brent Phillips
The Formula for Miracles – Where Science Meets Spirit
www.theformulaformiracles.com